Nourish

Nourish

A Modern Mother's Guide to Child Nutrition

Tamar N Henry

The content of this book is for general instruction only.
Each person's physical, emotional and spiritual condition is unique.
The instruction in this book is not intended to replace or interrupt the reader's
relationship with a physician or other professional.
Please consult your doctor for matters pertaining to your specific health and diet.

Matador
9 Priory Business Park,
Wistow Road, Kibworth Beauchamp,
Leicestershire. LE8 0RX
Tel: 0116 279 2299
Email: books@troubador.co.uk
Web: www.troubador.co.uk/matador
Twitter: @matadorbooks

ISBN 978 1788036 009

British Library Cataloguing in Publication Data.
A catalogue record for this book is available from the British Library.

Printed and bound by CPI Group (UK) Ltd, Croydon, CR0 4YY
Typeset in 11pt Adobe Garamond Pro by Troubador Publishing Ltd, Leicester, UK

Matador is an imprint of Troubador Publishing Ltd

Photography by Lindsay Lyon

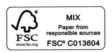

To mothers everywhere.

For my late Nanny Sylvia, my late Granny Christina,
my mother-in-law Therisita, my mother Linda,
my Aunty Susan and my sister Nikki
for your patience, your wisdom and for so much love.

Nourish
(verb)

1: To sustain with food or nutrient; to supply what is necessary for life, health and growth.

2: To cherish, foster and keep alive.

3: To strengthen.

Contents

Acknowledgements

Where would I be without my family? Without their unwavering love and support I would not have the motivation or resolve to stand steadfast on my principles and therefore my actions. Each and every one of them has always been there for me, to offer their encouragement, and for that I am eternally grateful.

My two grandmothers, who sadly have passed, offered me so much insight as I was growing up. I don't think I knew it then but I certainly do now. I think of them often and fondly, for their strengths, their wisdom and their home-made foods.

Thank you, thank you, thank you to my mother and father (Mum and Dad) for always being there for me. In a world where it seems it has become so difficult to stay healthy I remember a time where you made it look so easy. As we know, health isn't simply about what we eat but about the love we receive, the emotions we are allowed to show, and the safety that is provided for us; as parents you both went out of your way to make me feel secure enough to achieve anything I set my mind to. Thank you for always being so proud of me. I love you!

My in-laws are a huge pillar of strength and help for us, and because of them, I am being shown how to raise my boys in some non-traditional ways. My mother-in-law, having raised many children, knows only too well the patience, care and dedication it takes to nurture. As I watch her with my own boys my very real hope is that I can emulate her in some small way.

Dearest Aunty Susan, I just want to show gratitude to you, quite simply for being you. I have such fond memories of growing up spending time in your garden with the frogs and the snails. I think of summer when I think of you, of sunshine and of our Samantha. You are the archetype of growing old gracefully, full of beauty and boundless energy. I wish I saw you more.

Nikki, my sister, has been the one that I look up to. As my older sibling she has led the way, and has done so with such fierce determination and poise. As a paediatric nurse, it has been so reassuring to have her advice and expertise as we raise our young sons. I treasure our quality time together. Thank you Nikki (and not forgetting my brother-in-law Phil and my adorable nephew Harry) for loving and supporting me from afar.

Scott, my younger brother, I remember mothering you like you were my own. I'm not sure that I did a very good job at the time; being only six years older, but I think you will agree what great friends we became and still are.

Thank you to my dear friend Hayley, whom I have known all my life. I don't think there is a situation that we have not been through together. As a young mother to Casey I look back now and I realise how brave, strong and utterly determined you were to raise her right, and now she is the beautiful, confident young woman we see before us. Well done you!

My childhood friends, Gemma and Shelley, you are and always will be dear to me. You know all and everything that I am grateful to you for.

My Natasha, my Tashie, my Tash. Thank you for putting up with me for all these years. Nineteen years ago you took the only seat left in the classroom next to mine, and you have not left my side since. You are my confidante, my friend, and my beloved.

In my twenties, I got the opportunity to travel as I worked and some of those days were the best of my life. I have never talked so much about life's opportunities (sometimes all through the night) about what we might become. These girls, perhaps without knowing it, signalled a way for me to follow my dreams. I thank you, Charlotte, Claire, Jade, Nicola, and Sumi. Look, we made it, and look we are all mothers now!

For those dear friends who I can't forget and never will – we watched our babies grow side by side. Experiencing the start of motherhood together is something so special. Here's to many, many more years of seeing our families flourish! I thank you, Katee, Amy and Preet.

Thank you, Sophie, for giving me the confidence to stay home and raise my boys. You are inspirational as well as beautiful (inside and out), and your honesty is a gift only true friends can know.

Both professionally and personally, I want to thank my dear friend Aida, for your vision of creating a school where all children have the opportunity to learn about all aspects of health every day. Your school is quite simply an example of what schools should be. I thank you for giving me the freedom to teach with passion. Your kindness, integrity, and spirit are palpable, and I am truly blessed to know you.

Thank you, Hala, for allowing me to witness the inspired, strong and lovely woman that you are. Our time together, no matter how limited, was always inspiring.

Dr Ammer, I can never thank you enough for your expertise, professionalism and unrelenting care for Jul. I thank you for always taking the time to really listen to our concerns and for working 'with us' to provide health for all our children.

During some of the more difficult times with Jul I was fortunate enough to have friends that I could rely upon and depend. Cheryl, Kerri and Renee, I will not forget the time and devotion you gave to me.

To my friends who I have spent many years getting to know, Claire and Lindsay, our paths crossed once and I know they will again.

Alexis, I hope you know how special you and your family are to me. I look forward to a life long friendship with you.

To Erica, Heather, Jacqueline and Nancy, you may never know how your passion for doing what you love to do has encouraged me. I adore each one of you.

Janet, you have been so inspirational to me, as both a mother and friend. I thank you for your generosity and kindness. No matter where life takes us I know we will remain friends.

To those dear friends and neighbours, past and present, what a blessing to have each and every one of you in my life.

My children, my boys, I adore you, and I thank you for teaching me patience, unconditional love and the ability to go days without proper sleep! Grow healthy, my little ones, into the fine young men that I know you will be.

And lastly, gratitude must go to my husband, the father of my boys, my guide, and true north. Thank you for believing in me and for pushing me towards my dreams. L.O.V.E

Introduction

Jul

Nine years ago, I became a mother to my first son, Jul. He taught me to see the beauty in life where I had not seen it before, and yet, quite naturally, I also feared for my young child. As his mother, I was able to take care of his basic needs but I was about to find out it would take much more than this to keep him healthy.

A Mother's Intuition

Jul was born three weeks early, which made it difficult for me to nurse him right away. I suffered from complications due to the caesarean section, hence I felt pressured to bottle-feed. Despite my best efforts to provide Jul with breast milk, he was heavily supplemented with formula, which if I am honest, none of which ever really suited him. The skin on his face became inflamed, and he suffered from food allergies and hives. Although he was developing within the normal milestones, and in many ways was a perfectly happy baby, my intuition was that something was not quite right. At nine months old, our son became sick with viral meningitis, something I am happy to say that he recovered from, but over the next three years, he developed a variety of illnesses and symptoms that neither we as his parents, nor the doctors, understood. Our son, although bright and energetic, was not thriving as he should be, and as he celebrated his fourth birthday, our lives were turned upside down.

A simple throat infection turned out to be something much more sinister and after several routine checks by the doctor, we were referred to the children's ward of a local hospital. It was there that Jul, before our eyes began to bleed into his skin (petechiae), an alarming but common reaction to a drastically low red blood cell count. After several tests, a group of consultants asked to speak with us. Trying hard to understand all that was being said, we were given the terrifying news that Jul would have to be transferred by ambulance immediately and admitted to a children's oncology unit for suspected leukaemia.

A Parent's Worst Nightmare

In the ward, I vividly recall the noises: the machines, children crying in pain and discomfort, terrified parents doing all they could to lend some support. I attempted to block everything out. At twenty-eight weeks pregnant with our second son, I tried hard to remember my own health as well.

Over the course of the next few days, we would sit, wait and watch our sweet son in sorrow. Jul was terribly brave but started to stutter and then hardly spoke at all. The doctors told us this was a probable side effect of shock, and likely the result of all that was going on around him. After a trial blood transfusion that indicated no improvement, a bone marrow extraction had to be taken. It would be several hours later that day before the doctors were able to give us a definite diagnosis.

We were told Jul did *not* have leukaemia but a rather rare virus, Immune Thrombocytopenia (ITP), which he would, in time, recover from. My husband and I (although still visibly shaken) were elated. We could take our son home.

The weeks that followed were tense. Jul reacted well to the prescribed drugs, but with the improvement also came the side effects. He could do very little in terms of activity – not easy for a boy of his age, but Jul adapted well and fell in love with art. He would literally draw, sketch, colour and paint for hours (and still does).

Three months later and two weeks after the arrival of our second child, with no prior symptoms or warning, Jul was admitted to hospital again after waking with a sore throat diagnosed later that day as an abscess, which was threatening to cut off his airway. Jul became really sick, really fast. He was in a lot of pain, suffering from headaches and irritability, and I know from his actions, and as his mother, that he was scared. With the help from family and dear friends, either my husband or myself were able to be at our boy's side constantly. We lay with him, read to him, fed him, and all the while a battle raged on inside of him. Finally, after eight excruciating days, we all went home. Sigh…

Taking Matters Into My Own Hands

Even though I did not fully realise it at the time, the education that I was receiving through my studies towards a degree in health and wellness were lending me the confidence I needed to manage what we were going through. This self-assurance allowed me to be proactive with Jul's treatment and a forceful advocate for him. My husband and I didn't feel passive in this situation; on the contrary, we were committed participants in our son's recuperation, and I cannot tell you how important and necessary this is. As parents, we knew there had to be more to Jul's diagnosis, after everything he had gone through since infancy, and we were determined to find the answers. We were fortunate enough to be able to find a paediatrician in whom we put our trust, and from there, an immunologist and other specialists. Jul had (and will continue to have) an antibody deficiency, making it difficult when he gets sick for his body to heal. Through diet, close monitoring and support from his specialists, Jul is now, like any other active boy of his age. We have been told that his body has learned to cope with this deficiency, something that was more difficult at a younger age, and yet something we will continue to observe and work through.

A Time to Reflect

After our ordeal, and as I took the time to reflect, I realised any one of us can suffer ill health at any time. In Jul's case, he had a deficiency and there was little we could have done to prevent what he went through. Yet, I also know the medical care and attention he received, the devotion we provided for our child, and the education that I was pursuing (that is now my life's on-going work), were all real factors in Jul's improvement.

My Personal Mission

And so because of what Jul went through, what we went through as a family, I continued with my studies and became relentless in my pursuit of knowledge, thus learning more about health and nutrition and how to achieve and maintain it, and began to purposefully steer my family towards an optimal lifestyle. I think I realised at this point that for me, the challenges I faced within my own family could effectively help the lives of others. I began to see that certain nutrition principles could offer families the best opportunity to achieve health, and not as a means to heal only, but as a preventative for a better way of life.

As a practising health counsellor, I have become even more determined to set an example that others can follow. Nowadays, sadly, most health and nutrition advice is out-dated and/or misleading and lacks a clear foundation on the many aspects that are imperative to achieving lasting results. As I have personally experienced and seen in the homes of my many clients, health success is never the result of pure chance; it is with a driven purpose and sincere effort that accomplishments are made.

A Mother's Message

Life doesn't come with a manual; it comes with a mother.
(Anon)

As I continue to raise my three sons, now nine, five and two, I feel on a daily basis the extent to which I am personally responsible for our family's nutrition. Even as a health professional, I understand the enormity of this and how difficult it can be to learn the steps for necessary change and long-term maintenance.

While health encompasses many vital components, I feel confident in saying that holistic nutrition is key, and often the catalyst for all-round health.

Where should you begin, I hear you say?

NOURISH guides you through five focus points that may challenge your current concept of what it takes to achieve optimal nutrition, and to successfully nourish your family, in and outside of the home. Each focus point will introduce you to an approach that may be new to you. The information, and the real-life experiences that I write about, will slowly enhance your understanding, begin or further your education on this current topic, provide you with simple but effective methods to implement right away, and empower you so that transformation can happen.

Thus, it is my hope for each and every one of you that NOURISH makes its way into your busy homes, offering your family the chance to learn simple changes that lead to permanent results.

Featured in NOURISH – Words and Their Meanings

(Good for you to know!)

Additives – an ingredient added in order to improve or preserve e.g. essence, extract, flavouring).

Child – a blessing or precious being: the result of love: a little human you would walk the Earth for.

Deficient – not having enough of something that is necessary, defective, inadequate, lacking or poor.

Diet – the typical foods that a person routinely eats; their eating habits, pattern of eating, regime etc.

Food – a substance consisting of essential nutrients that humans need to live and grow; sustenance.

Free-range – poultry kept in more natural conditions, allowed to move about more freely, and access the outdoors.

GMO – genetically modified organisms (artificially manipulated, genetically engineered).

Health – the state of being well and/or free from illness or medical conditions; well-being; vigour.

Holistic – consideration of the whole person, complete, inclusive, whole.

Ingredient – one or more substances used to make a particular recipe; a small part of something bigger.

Junk food – processed, packaged, convenience food with little to no nutritional value; pre-prepared.

Lifestyle – the way in which a person chooses to live; a way of life; behaviours; a set of habits.

Longevity – living for many years; long existence/life.

Mother – a parent who is female, caring, instinctive and/or maternal.

Nutrient – a substance that provides nourishment; e.g. a nut contains many nutrients: fat, protein and vitamins.

Organic (fruits, vegetables, grains etc.) – foods produced by methods that comply with standards, grown free from artificial chemicals.

Organic (meats and dairy) – free from antibiotics; no GMO's; better treatment of animals.

Parenthood – the journey of raising your child; a huge commitment/mammoth undertaking.

Preservatives – a substance/chemical added to food to preserve life or prevent decay.

Processed – raw food that has been modified to taste different and last longer, containing additives.

Raw – food in its natural state: unaltered, uncooked and unprocessed.

Traditions – a belief or custom passed on from one generation to another; principles; a way of life.

Well-being – in a state of good health, comfortable, happy and well.

Wholefoods – foods that are unprocessed and unrefined, or as little as possible; no additives; whole.

Wholegrain – containing the whole grain, unprocessed and unrefined.

Chapter 1

FOCUS ON INDUSTRY

If we keep doing what we're doing,
we're going to keep getting what we're getting.
(Stephen R. Covey)

I have thought long and hard about what it will take for us
to realise the detrimental effects of foods that provide us with
little to no benefit, and the solution is to be informed. For it is
only when you know better, that you do better.

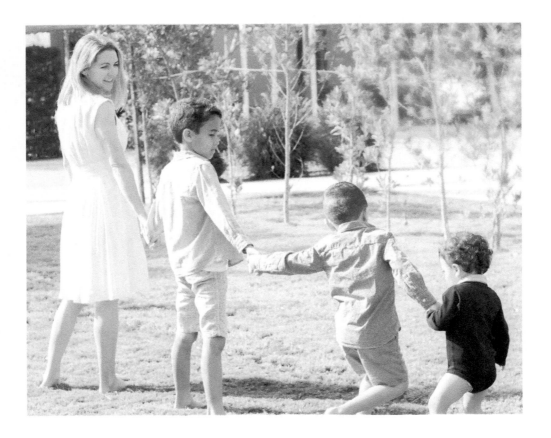

A Look at Life Around You

It is time to begin your journey into understanding the food industry and where what you eat comes from, but firstly I would like you to think about life, the world around you, your own community, with your extended family, maybe even in your own home, and seriously consider how food is failing health. We see, we read, and we hear about it all of the time, so much now that sadly, it has become commonplace to watch people suffer so unnecessarily. I think we all know someone, many people perhaps, who are battling ill health caused by poor diet, a sedentary lifestyle and/or a lack of health awareness. People are deteriorating at a much younger age from conditions driven by inadequate diet and weight gain. More children are impaired by food intolerances, from allergy symptoms and reactions, and their bodies are significantly compromised by harmful ingredients and substances added to their foods. Perhaps your own child is sick and you are unsure where to begin or how to get help.

I want to know about healthy foods because I really don't want to get fat,
most of all I really don't want to get sick.
(Student, aged eight and a half)

How Change Happened

I was brought up among a generation that has seen the most dramatic shift in where our food comes from and how it is produced, and although the change has been life-altering it is very likely that you didn't see it happening at all. So now, as parents to children of the new generation, who will continue to get sicker and more affected if we don't do something, it is imperative that we do see this, and that we bring about change quickly.

Things were definitely different when I was raising my children. I worried much
less about what to feed my family than I see young mothers doing now.
I feel very sorry for them.
(Linda, mother to children aged forty-two, thirty-eight and thirty-three)

Maybe your own childhood, more likely your parents and grandparents, was filled with memories of seeing animals living freely on farms – cattle had plenty of green grazing land, and poultry wide open spaces – and with appropriate nutrition. These animals were almost certainly tended to by skilled farmers, whose livelihood was passed down from one generation to another. This way of life was hard but sacred to these farmers. They seemed to care about the animals, just like the growers who tended to field upon field of crops and fruits and vegetables. This allowed you to eat local produce in season without harsh chemicals to produce them. Your parents would almost certainly have bought their meats from a butcher or straight from the farmer, their weekly fruits and vegetables from the local grocer. Your mother and hers were likely to have been very experienced in the kitchen, producing sumptuous and appetising foods, meal after meal, for the family. Convenience foods were not all that common, and if they were available, only eaten sparingly.

Fast-forward through my teenage years and into adulthood, and the presence of fast food, junk food; processed foods (what I like to call non-real foods) were evident. Yes, you could and can still buy everything that your typical diet was made up of, but the majority of your foods were and are no longer fundamentally the same.

There are still men and women who work the land determinedly to bring its customers products that are still cultivated in the same way all these years later, organic produce from natural agriculture that is uncontaminated, free of pesticides and chemicals, free of hormones and further additives. They have not relinquished their values and have not sold out to corporations, despite it being very difficult to stay profitable. You can find them, but they are much fewer than before, and unless you appreciate the true value of their work and produce you will more than likely shop elsewhere. It's important to understand that the alternative is going to be detrimental to your family's health.

Food Giants

Today, a large number of farms and farmers have been replaced by businesses and businessmen and women, overtaken and overrun by huge corporations. These giant companies make up the food industry (well, the large proportion that cares more about your money than your health, anyway) and this industry is not what you might know, or assume, or expect it to be. It spends enormous sums of money to misinform its consumers through dishonest advertising, misleading marketing, unproven health claims, false role models and wrongly labelling its products and ingredients.

> *I don't get it – why don't I know what's really going on?*
> *(Hala, aged eleven)*

Furthermore, the industry accepts and widely uses harmful substances, damaging to human health, in everyday foods, purchased unknowingly by well-intentioned parents (just like you and me) for their children. There is surplus evidence to prove a direct correlation between what we consume and our health, and yet in modern society it is made more difficult to eat well because of the constant hijacking of real foods that are so readily made available. Products commonly produced by these corporate giants have been farmed or produced using dangerous pesticides, mass-produced meat and dairy may include not only natural but artificial hormones, and all processed convenience foods include ingredients (or too much of one ingredient) that health professionals agree are not suitable for maximum nutrition, particularly in children: excess amounts of sugar, fats and salt, as well as a large number of additives: preservatives, artificial sweeteners, colourings, toxins, trans fats...

These corporations control a huge percentage of supermarket shelf space, meaning that the methods used to produce them, and the majority of ingredients they contain (many that you will be trying to eliminate), will be the same. This also means that if you do the bulk of your grocery shopping in supermarkets, locally sourced, better quality products will be more difficult to find.

Making a Change

If I could ask each of you individually if you know what you can do to be a trailblazer for better health for your family, would you say you do? Having the desire and passion to do more is easy, but having the dedication to follow through takes considerably more effort. There is only one sure way to demand quality foods (and it has been and is being done): only buy those products you know with certainty are nutritionally acceptable for your family. The only way to do this is to take a genuine interest in your family's food. Who makes it, where it comes from, and what it contains.

As your child's caretaker it is very possible for you to take the actions needed and take back the duty of raising your child on a nutritious diet, not just adequately but totally.

My health concerns about raising my young children are: am I giving them all the right nutrients for them to develop to the fullest? For them to be strong in mind, body and soul? I worry that even if I think I am giving them the correct foods, they might have been tampered with in some way. I worry that I don't fully understand the product information and if certain ingredients will hinder development, are

appropriate for a certain age, or even if all the information is being put onto the label in the first place!
(Nancy, mother to children aged three and one)

Harmful Substances

Pesticides – in order to kill nuisances such as weeds and bugs to keep from destroying or delaying the natural growing processes of agriculture, some farming practices use toxic substances that pollute the immediate and surrounding environment. Contamination of food by pesticides is very dangerous, and the more foods you eat containing toxins, the more harmful to your health it is.

Artificial Hormones – in some countries the non-organic farming industry regularly uses artificial hormones in animals that are produced for meat and/or dairy. The unnatural method of injecting artificial hormones is used to increase weight in animals for more meat, and in dairy cows to increase milk production. For both the animal and for us consuming its products, the increased exposure to oestrogen is damaging to health.

Sugar – it is widely accepted that sugar is a substance with addictive potential. Therefore, dependency on sugar caused by eating too much of it can have serious implications for your child's health. The recommended amount of added sugar (sugar not sourced directly from natural foods, fruit for example) is only around five teaspoons per day.

Fats – eating fat is an essential part of any diet, however there are two types, non-saturated (considered healthy to eat) and saturated (recommended to eat in lower amounts as it can contribute to high cholesterol, heart disease and other diet-related illnesses). Healthy fats can be found in avocado, some nuts and seeds, olive oil, oily fish and soya beans. Less healthy, saturated fats are found in dairy products, meat and processed oils.

Salt – too much sodium elevates a person's blood pressure, resulting in increased levels of fluid in the body. Too much salt is linked to a number of life-threatening diseases. Processed foods contain large amounts of salt and should be avoided where possible for your family. Cut back on adding salt to your children's meals, and if needed add authentic sea salt at the table. Natural sea salt contains a number of essential elements from the sea that in small amounts are good for us.

Additives – food additives are substances used to help preserve the shelf life, taste and/or appearance of food. Some food additives have been used for centuries, are considered healthful and include vinegar, natural salts and vitamin C, however more recently, cheaper, long-lasting substances have been used as replacements, meaning companies can produce food that looks better for longer, for less money. The obvious compromise for the consumer is that in order to enjoy such foods, your health could be seriously at risk.

The most commonly used food additives are sadly the ones that are doing us the most harm, causing headaches, nausea, vomiting, irritability, mood swings, allergy symptoms and reactions, and when ingested regularly can contribute to chronic diseases. Although these additives may not be familiar to you right now, they are easy to identify because of the unusual names or numbers given to them, either difficult to pronounce or to spell, on food labels. Here I list the top ten:

Aspartame (E951)
An artificial sweetener (to which brands often give another name) is widely used in sugar-free or diet products.

High Fructose Corn Syrup (HFCS)
Found in a majority of processed products, known to easily cause weight gain and increase levels of bad cholesterol.

Monosodium Glutamate (MSG; E621)
Commonly added to takeaway foods, snack items and particular brands of stock cubes, MSG is used to enhance flavour.

Trans Fats
When manufactured, trans fats are also known as partially hydrogenated oils. Among health professionals trans fats are believed to be the worst type of fat you can consume. Mostly found in margarine and baked and fried foods.

Food Dyes
The worst offenders (blue #1, blue #2, red #3, red #40, yellow #6, yellow tartazine or E102) are banned in some European countries. Also known as artificial colourings, food dyes are frequently found in cereals, some cheeses, ice cream, salad dressings, sweets, soft drinks and fruit juices, and have been strongly linked to behavioural issues in children.

Sodium Sulphite (E221)

Used mostly to preserve dried fruits, sulphites have the potential to cause allergy-like effects – asthma symptoms are the most reported symptoms in people with an underlying condition. Sulphites can also cause wheezing, hives, and in rare and extreme cases even anaphylaxis (a reaction that can cut off your airway entirely, needing urgent medical care).

Sodium Nitrate/Sodium Nitrite

Used in different types of processed meat and fish, sodium nitrate is used to colour, flavour and preserve. When consumed it can be carcinogenic (cancer-causing).

BHA/BHT (E320)

These offenders are used to prevent food containing fats and oils from going bad, and are commonly found in cereal, crisps and sweets.

Sulphur Dioxide (E320)

Found mostly in soft drinks, juices and vinegar, sulphur dioxide is toxic. Not recommended for children, sulphur dioxide can cause allergy-like reactions and symptoms, mild and severe.

Potassium Bromate

In many countries potassium bromate is banned for use in foods although in others it is commonly used as a flour enhancer. Found in breads.
(Source: Food Matters).

If you worry that your family is consuming some of the additives listed here, please take a closer look at product packaging to find out, and where possible avoid them altogether or find healthier alternatives – they are out there. (Better still, be inspired in the next chapter and make your own!)

Something to Think About
Your children are unique and will respond in their own way to different substances, so consider additives when you notice unusual symptoms.

I grew up having migraines, a condition which is often brought on or worsened by processed foods, so it wasn't until my mother was told to keep a food diary that she could link my symptoms to specific foods and modify my diet accordingly. Furthermore, it wasn't until I realised that ordinary bags of dried apricots that I was regularly purchasing were the likely cause of one of my son's allergy symptoms that I thought to link the issue to the additive sodium sulphate, which at the time I didn't have any idea was potentially so harmful.

I find it really hard to believe that these substances, toxic and harmful, are not more commonly understood, more thoroughly regulated, better labelled, and in some cases banned altogether.

> *Why are companies allowed to get away with this stuff? Why are they allowed to make food that is no good for us? I don't understand – shouldn't they be in trouble or something?*
> *(Student, aged eight)*

Transitioning to eating better can take some time, however it is never too soon to eradicate the most harmful offenders from your family's diet. Below are some instant ways to help you select quality food choices, and it's recommended that you speak about these with your children:

Don't eat anything you don't immediately recognise as food.

This may be difficult for our children's generation, as they are so used to seeing so many processed foods. Help them to decipher which products are real and which are not. (An apple is real; a toffee apple is not. Potatoes are nutritious; deep-fried chips are not. Fresh fruits are loaded with vital vitamins; fruit flavoured products are not.) Notice that although some products lead you to believe, through the pictures and words on their packaging that they include a particular fruit or vegetable, most don't. When you inspect the ingredients list you find there is no sign of a single fruit or vegetable, just artificial colourings and preservatives. This is commonly seen in cereals, confectionery, desserts, ice cream and sweetened yoghurts.

Don't buy anything if you don't know what it contains.

If a product seems identifiable to you as a real food, but you are still unsure because perhaps it is spiced, sugared, crumbed or coated, do take the time to quickly scan through the ingredients list. If on closer inspection you don't recognise the substances, or the list is extensive and/or incomprehensible, then it is very likely you are looking at some of the additives that you are aiming to avoid.

Don't pick products that are brightly coloured.
All children are drawn to bright colours and manufacturers of foods and drinks
know this. Only those foods derived from nature (think fruits and vegetables)
have a colour that is both radiant and nutritious. Unless a product is specified
as containing natural colours originating from fresh fruit or vegetable juices,
it most certainly contains artificial dyes that will be detrimental to both your
child's short- and long-term health.

Don't buy anything you can make yourself.
Some foods, when purchased and stored correctly, will retain their freshness and
taste despite having a long expiry date. This will be the case for many of your
pantry items – think rice, pasta, flour, beans, nuts, seeds and oils. Items such as
salad dressings, sauces, boxed juices and even packaged bakery items etc. have a
scarily long time before they expire, but only because of the additives that they
contain. Think about it: if you make any of these items yourself, they will last
only one to seven days (even if refrigerated) before going bad. Commercially
prepared salad dressings, for example, despite ingredients such as oil and vinegar
that would naturally separate (but don't), do not expire as quickly, because of
the stabilisers and preservatives the manufacturers add. You may not know it
yet, but making more of your staple foods from scratch will in the long run save
you money, increase your child's health, and furthermore, as you will notice for
yourself, taste superior and be more satisfying.

Strategies for Change:
- Research current food standards for where you live. The differences between one
  country and another, even one region and another, might be significant.
- Find out where you can locally source more of your family's foods and ingredients.
- Start to familiarise yourself with the food industry, watch documentaries as a
  family, and read books and articles relating to topics of interest. Get informed. (See
  Resources and Recommendations).

Beware of Brands

As you begin to sit up and take notice of where your food comes from, you will unavoidably start to notice brands, the ones that are owned by the giant corporations we have been talking about. They are everywhere. It may seem at first that you are being bombarded from every angle: the Internet, television, commercials, street advertising, marketing literature handed out or put through your door, promotions at concerts and social events, even school textbooks and children's books, and of course at the supermarket. Yet it has always been there, cleverly and oh-so-carefully creeping into your life as if it were a normal part of it. This is, as you might expect, what the retailers want.

> *Outside influences and external forces can provide challenges in maintaining standards or expectations that are observed within the home. As my eldest child is growing he is more likely to be influenced by advertising, however as we have instilled good routines and habits around food*
> *I hope this will help him to continue to make good choices.*
> *(Charlotte, mother to children aged six and three)*

In order to raise your child as much as possible in a processed-free world, it will be up to you to avoid where possible Internet applications made for kids that allow junk food advertising, to abstain from buying big brands for your kitchen and home, to distract or deter your children away from convenience foods when out and about, and as I talk passionately about in Chapter 3, to educate them to know better.

The Internet

Now that Jul is using his computer and the Internet more for schoolwork I have become more aware of what he might now be exposed to. I had expected that some convenience foods would be marketed online, but what I didn't expect was just how many would be. I also wasn't aware (and maybe you are not also) that although he may be researching for or watching something that is entirely age-appropriate, that the ads that lead or follow on from this material are at times not. Now I find myself worrying about his Internet usage, and checking every application, even those recommended and labelled as 'educational', to see what other unhealthy habits they may encourage.

I am further agitated by kids' apps (those my middle son likes) that I hoped would be a safer, healthier platform for him to enjoy. He has learned so much over the years when watching nursery rhymes and songs, and other educational videos to learn his numbers, counting, how to spell etc., and of course I have picked out those ones that have taught him where his food comes from, farming, fruits and vegetables, healthy cooking etc., and so I have been really disappointed lately to see videos displaying kid after kid eating convenience foods, in particular sweets. Although the standards promise that no paid advertising for food brands will be allowed, uploaded amateur videos that show exactly this type of exposure are. I have to tell you I have been a little repulsed and very confused by the trend that shows clips of children unwrapping, licking and/or eating junk! Is it really too much to ask that a forum dedicated to our growing children prevents such videos that sneakily advertise and glamorise junk food, something which we all know to be so detrimental to children's health? Surely, we can do better than this?

> *I tend not to buy unhealthy brands, because if I did then my children would be exposed to them and that's not my intention. I make sure to keep cupboards and the fridge well stocked with a variety of alternatives. I bake bread and muffins, make muesli bars and the like, and allow my kids to take turns in choosing what I make. I think it's important for them to learn about nutrition also, and for them to hear about what's in their food and understand what ingredients (good and bad) do to their body. When we lived in our previous home we really loved growing vegetables, and taking part in the entire process meant the children ate them eagerly.*
> *(Janet, mother to children aged twelve, nine and three)*

Public Places

If you choose to dine out in an Italian restaurant then you will expect to eat Italian food, and if I want sushi I won't go to a burger bar. What I am surprised to get, however, whenever I take my children out, is the over abundance of convenience foods that are a concoction of high fructose corn syrup, surplus sugars and salts, and too many additives, preservatives and artificial colours to mention. Is it too much to expect that the places that are purposely built for our growing children to partake in physical activities and play can offer them anything more than unwholesome food?

> *Kids are not really made to eat any kind of junk food, and so it*
> *makes me mad to see so much of it everywhere you go.*
> *(Student, aged eight)*

As a mother to three young sons I cannot tell you the countless times that I have been to a children's indoor play park, recreation centre or specifically themed activity area and been sorely disappointed by the food options my children have been presented with. Yes, you can find (if you look hard enough) the occasional baked potato, small salad and a bottle of water, but that's about it among the vending machines and the array of fried foods, sandwiches made with white bread, crisps, cakes (so, so many cakes!) sweetened yoghurts, a vast array of chocolate bars, processed soft drinks, fizzy drinks, energy drinks – the list goes on (as you will certainly have seen for yourself). If you do not frequent these spots all that often and you tire of packing your own food to take absolutely everywhere for your child, then I understand your yearning to turn a blind eye, but I plead with you not to.

The problem only worsens when we continue to do so, and the endless cycle of food that is no good for our children is constantly supplied and offered. Just like the foods you are trying to avoid in the supermarket, if you don't buy them, eventually they won't sell them and your demand for other foods will take precedence. It might be difficult at first but if you feel strongly enough then it is time to stop eating in such places, make your complaints (nicely), and opt to bring your own food instead. If enough people did this, I can assure you the management would change their menus rather than suffer a lack of profit.

My sincere hope for the future is that no location that directly caters for children's play, or places dedicated to sports and other life-enhancing pursuits, targets consumers with non-nutritious food and drink. Let us dare to dream how pleasurable it would be to be able to say yes to any food request that our child makes. Imagine the lack of drama and the increased amount of time your child and their friends would have to play because no one is having a meltdown because someone else is eating something which you have declared they cannot eat (because after all that would be undermining everything you stand for and that is good for them), or because they have had their weekly recommended amount of sugar in just one afternoon! I digress, but wouldn't it be lovely?

> *I see other mothers giving their children junk food and they seem OK, but then I think*
> *maybe they are having just as hard a time as I am feeding their child well, and when*
> *they are out they just don't know what to choose. It's hard.*
> *(Hayley, mother to children aged five and one)*

Poor Role Models

As I discuss in depth in Chapter 5, you are an essential role model for your child, but what about the power of outside influences? From a really young age children are highly impressionable and prone to mimicking those people and behaviours they are exposed to the most. Whether we like it or not, our children pick up habits that may not be in line with the principles we are trying to impart. As a parent, this can be difficult to contend with.

When it comes to what your child learns about the food they will use to fuel their body, the health and food industries will play a major part. Despite all the good that is being done in engaging our youth in health education and physical activities, and the many ad campaigns that we see to prevent ill health, they cannot compete with the enormous sums of money which are being used to promote non-nutritious food and drink, and I cannot help but be incredibly frustrated by this. I am also concerned about the hugely famous celebrities who are willing to endorse such products.

> *When I see someone who I thought was a good role model being unhealthy I feel that instead of showing me what I should be doing, they are now showing me what I shouldn't.*
> *(Nicky, aged ten)*

Today, our children are very much part of a generation that wrongly or rightly is directly manipulated by the celebrity culture. As parents it is of course up to us to steer our children towards only that which is age-appropriate in terms of the TV they're watching or the types of celebrity they are following, but what about those we very much see as a positive influence, a healthy role model, those who positively impact and increase participation in physical activity and eating better? What then are we to do as parents, if we are already disappointed with the lack of integrity shown by most major brands that we are trying to avoid, when celebrities with a huge youth following, particularly sports men and women, are happy to endorse them? Obviously they do this for more money and fame, but it is hugely disappointing coming from someone who is a positive influence for children, and a massive contradiction to what they generally stand for.

Something to Think About

I have done my research and almost every food and drink endorsed by a celebrity is unhealthy, and in most cases is commonly considered a junk food: fast food, sweets and soft drinks (all overly processed, lacking nutrients and for the most part sugary).

If I saw my idol being unhealthy I would feel bad for them, that they had this amazing talent that they had put out into the world and are then hurting themselves.
(Student, aged ten)

Strategies for Change:

- Prevent brand exposure by removing all foods from their boxes, cartons and wrappers. Place the food item in clear packaging or on the plate for your family. Get your child used to the idea that food does not always come from a packet, despite the fact that it may be healthy.
- Prevent brand exposure in your home, and on your child's plate or in their snack box, by providing more home-made foods.
- When out and about, limit your experiences with brands by bringing your own food and drinks.

Supermarket Shopping

The supermarket can be a daunting place to shop, especially if you are seeking to find produce that will support your family's health. Most major chains house over thirty thousand products, often making it difficult and time-consuming to find what you are searching for. However, current demand for superior produce means that quality products are now available, as long as you know what you are looking for and where in the supermarket to find them.

> *The fact that you really have to stop and search (and research) while in the supermarket is frustrating and time-consuming. If we knew all the options available to us were safe, then grocery shopping would be much more enjoyable. I'm a single working mum and honestly I don't have the excess time that grocery shopping sometimes demands. I worry that although I think I am making the right choices, I am probably not doing as well as I could be.*
> *(Mandy, mother to daughter aged twelve)*

Popular brands (those that are less likely to be good for you) tend to monopolise supermarket shelf space. Major corporations pay more money for more space, and for precise positions that easily catch the eye of the consumer. For some products, multiple displays are made of the same item; then strategically placed in various places around the store (think soft drinks), making it more probable that customers will end up buying this product, even if they didn't set out to do so. These retailer tactics are what cause most of our impulse buying when roaming the aisles. Try not to go to the supermarket without a precise shopping list. Buy only those items you know you absolutely need and that are necessary, and this will save you a lot of time and help you to avoid unfamiliar foods that you might hastily pick up and want to try.

For your children the hardest part of supermarket shopping will almost certainly be checking out, where a whole host of confectionery will be waiting for them, and this is why so many mums dread taking their child grocery shopping in the first place. Even if you have done an incredible job of keeping your child distracted from other non-nutritious foods around the store, it is pretty much impossible to avoid in the check-out queue unless you have someone with you who can successfully distract or take your child outside. Admittedly, even those children who know all too well that these are not good choices will be tempted to look and to ask for them. This is the time where if you do give in, like everything else, your child will expect it the next time and the time after that, and so on and so on, making it difficult for you, to ever break the habit. On the rare occasion when I do take my boys supermarket shopping with me I usually have a healthy snack in my bag that I pull out for them at this time; perhaps a home-made cookie or muffin or an all-fruit-juice lollipop, something appealing enough to divert them away from all the processed food.

After reading NOURISH in its entirety I very much hope that you will consider what you buy for your family much more carefully. I feel confident that you will start making more of your family's foods, knowing exactly what products you will need and the best way to source them. You will start to consider local shops and online resources as a way to seek out the right products for your home, which will make repeat buying (and not having to look endlessly for new products) such a relief. I can honestly tell you that for the past five years or more I have been buying the same things even though I am making an array of menus to feed my family.

One of my services as a health counsellor is 'the health food store tour', which allows me to guide clients around the supermarket, avoiding as much as possible the aisles and products that are not necessary in their family's diet or lifestyle. My clients also receive the hands-on guidance in how to detect harmful ingredients and how to read food packaging and labels properly. What people are surprised to find out is that by staying on the periphery of a supermarket (as they are all pretty much designed with the same layout), you will find most of the items you will need: your fresh produce (fruits, vegetables and herbs), nuts, seeds and dried fruits, the bakery section, meats and dairy. Of course you will need to stock up on pantry items every month or so, but the bulk of your shop can be done quickly, and with avoidance of the endless aisles of merchandise with little to no nutritional value.

The Healthy Brands

It can be a little difficult at first to differentiate the healthy brands from the non-nutritious ones. What may help you initially is looking for the packaged foods that you normally purchase (crackers, cereals etc.) in the organic aisle. Supermarkets may not always do a great job of separating items, but in general this aisle contains produce that is notably less processed, that offers higher nutrition content and that adheres to organic rules and regulations. Once you become adept at reading food labels, finding what you want will become easier.

Age-Appropriate

This may certainly seem like a new concept to some, but ensuring that your child is eating the appropriate foods for their age is important. For the first year of a baby's life we are careful to nourish our child with the recommended amounts and types of milk and starter foods they need. We continue to chop or slice up foods that we deem dangerous to be eaten in their entirety (think grapes) and, withhold from offering our young child what we consider to be adult food. Yet as the years go by we can become careless (and let's face it, busy), and sincerely unawares as to what foods are best for our child at each stage. Think about it: just because your two-year-old now has the mobility to roam around the supermarket or take from your plate, doesn't mean he or she should pick up, open and/or be able to eat the first thing they find. Processed items particularly, are likely to contain too much salt, have spices he or she has not yet been exposed to yet, and possibly a host of unnecessary preservatives and colourings.

All foods that are processed (anything in a bottle, box, jar or packet, unless specifically detailed otherwise) will contain some form of preservative in order to give them shelf life. Each product will vary in its ingredients, some of which will be unsuitable for young children. I ask you to be particularly watchful for products you may now be looking for as your child reaches its toddler years, that may contain large amounts of sugar and salt: biscuits, cereals, crisps, crackers, soft drinks, flavoured yoghurts, even stock cubes. Making your own (or seeking out brands you know and trust) where possible is still more beneficial for children of this age.

Something to Think About

A lot of food and beverages because of the ingredients they contain, are not suitable for anyone, no matter our age. Those products that contain nasty additives, those that you are learning are no good for your child, are also no good for you. Try not to get into the habit of claiming that certain foods and drinks are for adults only. Stating so will only make them more appealing. If you can, avoid these foods and drinks altogether and furthermore refrain from having them in the house.

Children's Foods

I have to admit that I am deeply offended, highly frustrated and genuinely disappointed when a product that claims to be healthy turns out not to be, especially those targeted at children! For this reason I am thrilled with the many honest, well-intentioned companies that do a fabulous job of choosing more wholesome ingredients to preserve their goods. Cherry-pick these products by seeking recommendations from friends, enquire about the brand yourself, and buy only from those that you can trust to help feed your family.

The majority of reliable brands were created by mums and dads (just like you and me), who were frustrated by what the food industry had to offer and wanted to provide something more for their children and others. I applaud them and I am glad that they exist for those parents looking for a little bit of convenience in their already very busy lives.

> *I stopped eating lollipops and I missed them at first, but my mum found healthier alternatives and now I'm OK with not having the ones that my friends are eating – mine taste better and don't leave colour all over my mouth and tongue!*
> *(Student, aged eight)*

These goods, although packaged, are overflowing with goodness and created very specifically with children and their young taste buds in mind. Some of my favourites have no sugar added – *e.g.* organic cereal, fruit bars and purees. Unlike corporate brands that shamelessly use false marketing and tactics to try to conceal what's inside, trustworthy organic brands promote the healthy ingredients they contain. I love the fact that I can present my boys with something bright and appealing without compromising their health.

Success at the Supermarket

Prepare your child for the supermarket just as you would for a party or any other event where there may be foods that are less than desirable. Expect that the supermarket will present unhealthy food items that will be very appealing to the young child. If possible, don't let your child enter the supermarket hungry – as adults we know all too well the temptations that lurk within that are suddenly appealing when we are peckish. Talk with your child about what foods you will be looking for, encourage them to help out, and if you can shop on the periphery of the supermarket as recommended, avoiding the brightly coloured, processed items that will so easily entice your child.

As you motivate yourself further and make a real effort not to be put off by the massive food companies and their endless marketing, and as it becomes easier to navigate your way through the supermarket and questionable food labels, and as you search to find those trusted local businesses and their produce, you will start to enjoy a more fulfilling shopping experience (and the kids will too).

Non-Food Brands

Just as cautiously as I am asking you to consider what your family puts into their mouths, I am requesting also that you consider those products that you are using as part of your child's skincare, hair care and oral hygiene routines as well. Toothpaste, soap, baby wash, shampoo, oil, moisturiser and sunscreen can all play havoc with your child's skin and overall health if not sought out with knowledge of what you are looking for. Once again, one would very much hope to expect that those products purposely created for children would not contain harsh chemicals and preservatives, but very sadly a lot of them do. The best advice I can give you here is to buy 100% organic (or as near to as you can). There are some super companies offering really effective results, and the money you will pay will be worth it once you find them, treasure them and repeat buy. For more information on brands that I have personally sought out and use for my family, please see Resources and Recommendations.

If you are still unsure, need further clarification or want personal recommendations for your child or family (especially if one or more of your family have dietary issues, a skin complaint, or condition, or suffer from allergies) do seek out a holistic health professional who can help you with this. One of my busiest roles (and one of my favourites) is helping mothers to find products that really work for their family's individual needs (because I truly know how excruciating it can be to not find success with over-the-counter or prescription products). After years of researching companies and their products I have an unbiased list of products that I feel comfortable sharing. Once you try these items and they work for your family, you may never need to use other potentially harmful, perhaps even medicinal items again. As a mother who went from dermatologist to dermatologist looking for a cure for eczema caused by the climate we live in, I was finally able to abate the swelling, pain and irritation in a matter of a few short days, and prevent my other children (and so many more) from having to go through the same.

Strategies for Change:

- Set realistic expectations for your children before entering the supermarket. Talk about what they will do and what they will not do. Clear expectations provide your child with the probability that they will cooperate more.
- When making your shopping list, think about the food items that will be easy for your child to look for and depending on their age, make it a game or task. My boys love picking out exact numbers of the specific types of fruits and vegetables that we need.
- Seek out the perfect groceries, pantry items and self-care products for your family and repeat buy. The amount of time and effort this will save you will be profound.

Children's Comments: Aged Five to Ten.

How difficult is it for you to go to the supermarket and avoid unhealthy food items?
Some people I know say it's difficult to go to the supermarket and I understand why because of all the bright packaging and sweet foods they might want to eat, but for me it's easy, but only because I have learned about the dangers of eating them. At home, at school and on my own I am looking for information that stops me eating such gross food. (Student, aged nine)

What's the hardest part about being in a supermarket?
I feel bad when I see all the sweets and I can't have them. I wish they weren't there. (Sahm, aged five and a half)

Can you tell the difference between foods that are nutritious and those that are not?
Junk food tastes and feels weird in my mouth. I can tell almost instantly that it is not natural. Now that I am old enough to know better, and mostly because I am interested in staying healthy, I have learned to look for foods that are not good for me and know what they can do to my body, and because of this I don't want such food any more. (Student, aged ten)

Why do you think it's important to know where your food comes from and how it affects the body?
I think it's really important and I like learning the different ways to keep my body healthy. I think I should know what is in my food. Sometimes it's still hard for me to choose good foods but the more I learn, the easier it is – I can do it! (Student, aged seven and three quarters)

What motivates you to be healthy?
I see some of my family members who are overweight and I don't want to be like that, not ever. This is why I like doing sports, I like a lot of them, and why I like learning about how to be fit in school, and from sportspeople I watch on TV and, from my brothers. (Student, aged eight)

Do you prefer going to the supermarket or the local market?

I don't really like going to the supermarket as it seems to take so long to shop there. I also notice that there are so many foods that we don't eat there and I'm sure it would be difficult to choose even if we did. I like it a lot more going to farmers' markets and local shops as pretty much everything there I can try and a lot of things we buy. My brothers and me enjoy picking out the fruits and vegetables here also, and because of this we know a lot of their names and how they are grown. (Jul, aged nine and a half)

Do you feel you are missing out on foods you are encouraged not to eat?

Not really, no. I do eat these foods once in a while and I don't think I really like them, not eaten regularly anyway. I know for sure, if I eat too much then I don't feel well. I really love beef burgers but not the ones from fast food restaurants, they hardly taste like real meat at all. I think because my mum has taught me the difference, making healthy choices has become much easier for me. (Student, aged eight)

Industry – Your Questions Answered

How have I been so completely unaware of how drastically the food industry has changed?

Quite honestly, we don't often know because the food industry doesn't want you to know. Food is packaged and marketed amazingly well, leaving little room to doubt the product or the fact that it may have been altered so much. Groceries that you have been buying for years (even those you had as a child), produced by brands that you thought you could trust, may over time have been seriously modified, but you haven't noticed or even thought to look at current standards or the ingredients lists. It only becomes obvious when you hear something, or if you are personally affected by it, or if you take the time to pursue the evidence and information for yourself. Without this, it is challenging to understand how profoundly things have changed.

Junk food is sometimes shown in my children's cartoons – how can I ever hope to avoid this exposure for my child?

Just like you did, your child will grow up in an imperfect world. There will always be something that as a parent you will need to distract your child from, but I believe what is more beneficial is to educate and inform him or her so that they understand what is going on around them and how to go about making better choices for themselves. With that being said, I am just as disappointed as you are that some of the more popular children's animated programmes show their characters liking or eating non-nutritious foods. In our home, because I have learned to make healthy alternatives to junk foods that still feel like a treat, I don't feel that my children are as affected by what they see compared with others who might insist on eating these foods because they want to imitate what they have seen.

I recently welcomed my first child and was surprised when a popular baby's skincare product reacted badly on my newborn's skin. I have no idea why this happened or what to use instead.

Just because a product has been on the market for many years, and has big brand exposure and a huge following doesn't mean it's good or good enough for your family. Babies are fragile, delicate little beings and should be treated as such, and if you knew what harmful substances are contained in many of these products you would likely be horrified. Just as you will be careful not to feed your child anything that is not suitable for him or her at this age, I recommend you do the same with all other products. Look for organic, gentler, safer, baby-specific ranges.

Chapter 2

FOCUS ON FOOD

Let food be thy medicine and medicine be thy food.

(Hippocrates)

There is a saying that 'nothing tastes as good as healthy feels'. If you have ever truly felt the energy, vitality and zest for life you get from eating well, you will know this to be true and if you haven't, wouldn't you want to, for your children? For your family? I witness all too often that people have a misconception that sustained health through wholefoods is unobtainable; that it takes too much hard work and is too difficult to maintain.

I am here to tell you that it is absolutely possible, and that through small yet consistent efforts, you and your family will be rewarded in more ways than you could have ever imagined.

What you eat or don't eat plays a major role in your health.
(Mark Hyman, MD)

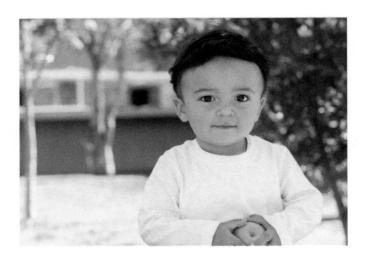

Eat Whole Foods

It sounds simple enough, doesn't it? Yet after everything we have learned about the food industry I think you will agree that choosing foods, to provide for your family takes consideration. Whole foods are foods from nature; that have not been altered significantly from their original state. These foods should make up a high percentage of your daily diet and include fresh fruits and vegetables, nuts, seeds, herbs, grains, and legumes. Fresh produce, where possible, should be organically farmed and locally and seasonally grown.

My mother, who is now sixty-four, told me constantly as a child, 'Don't eat anything against the law of nature, if you do it will have side effects'. Now that I am older and raising my own children in a vastly different time I realise the great importance of her message.
(Sarah, mother to children aged four and five)

Organic

Organic foods are grown and certified according to a country or region's governing body of set standards and procedures. The process of organic farming operates free from pesticides, herbicides, chemical fertilisers and genetically modified organisms, and does not involve further treatment by irradiation or food additives. If you are not aware of the harmful side effects of eating foods that are not manufactured organically, see Chapter 1 for more information. The very least you should know is that it puts extra strain on the immune system, weakening the body as a whole.

Meat and Dairy

If you do choose to feed your family products derived from meat and dairy, buy locally, from a farmer or source that you trust. Where possible, look for products that are organic *and* free-range (eggs), organic *and* grass-fed (cattle), and organic *and* pasture-raised (poultry and pork).

As a family, we view organic products as a way of ensuring the quality of the foods we consume. With so many different types of packaging and marketing gimmicks, it seems easier to go back to eating basic foods.
(Leigh, mother to children aged eight and five)

While the term 'organic' is commonly used, I fear consumers considerably underestimate the benefits of its produce, questioning whether the additional costs are worth it. With more accessibility than ever before, however, organic food can be found easily. You don't necessarily have to travel to your nearest farm shop or market (although I have to tell you it's well worth it), because organic aisles can be found at your local supermarket.

Something to Think About

As you become more aware of your health, and begin to think about nutrition for your family, you will surely add more fresh and wholefoods to your diet. Shopping organically, therefore, is something to consider seriously.

If you are still not sold on the idea of buying organic foods, think about it at least for produce that tops the 'Dirty Dozen' list. These fruits and vegetables, according to the Environmental Working Group, are those that contain the highest level of contamination through the conventional farming process.

Although the 'Clean Fifteen' may still be conventionally grown, these fruits and vegetables are considered to be at less risk for contamination, making them a healthier, more cost-effective choice when available and in season.

Shopper's Guide to Pesticides in Produce

The Dirty Dozen (buy these organic)	The Clean Fifteen (lower in pesticides)
1. Celery	1. Onions
2. Peaches	2. Avocado
3. Strawberries	3. Sweetcorn
4. Apples	4. Pineapple
5. Blueberries	5. Mango
6. Nectarines	6. Sweetpeas
7. Bell Peppers	7. Asparagus
8. Spinach	8. Kiwi
9. Cherries	9. Cabbage

10. Kale/collard greens
11. Potatoes
12. Grapes (imported)

10. Aubergine/Eggplant
11. Melon/Cantaloupe
12. Watermelon
13. Grapefruit
14. Sweet potato
15. Honeydew melon

(Source: Environmental Working Group)

Buy Local

Locally grown produce enhances our health. When foods are produced close to your home, without harmful pesticides and chemicals, in a region and climate where they naturally grow, one can rely on these environmentally conscious foods that will add to your family's well-being.

Buying locally grown foods also supports your local farmer and not the massive corporations working strictly for profit and commercial purposes. Your buying power will keep local farmers in business, meaning quality food for you and your family for many years to come.

> *When I lived in Malta my family ate nearly all organically farmed vegetables, all locally sourced fruit and also wild fish. I was proud of the commitment that I made to feeding them well and the obvious investment in their future health. I can honestly say I felt joy when I placed their plates in front of them.*
> *(Erica, mother to children age six, four and two)*

Eat Seasonal

If you have ever eaten a handful of sweet and succulent strawberries picked right from the plant, or enjoyed the rich creaminess of a freshly baked sweet potato, you would have likely appreciated produce in season.

Eating both locally and seasonally is better for the economy, lighter on your wallet and kinder to the body. Of course, local produce may still be farmed and manufactured in a way that you are not comfortable with and so you may still feel the need to choose organic options, but you can be assured that fresh foods have not gone through the lengthy processes that are necessary for long-distance import.

For my part, I love buying local and seasonal produce, as it chooses my recipes for me. Pumpkin, for example, is not available locally in the summer months because it is more of a warming food and thus not required at this time for an optimal diet. Cucumbers, tomatoes, celery and the like are, however, more cooling foods, and so a salad made up of these options will better suit my family's needs during the warmer months.

Taste Matters

For my needs and my family's, taste is everything. If the goods I purchase and prepare are as nutritious and delicious as they can be, even those picky eaters among my family will succumb. When food has not been produced locally, this means it could have been transported from almost anywhere in the world, and taste among other aspects has been seriously compromised.

> *I became interested in making my family fresh juice after I read how beneficial it could be. I started out in a country where it was difficult to find local, let alone organic produce, but I made do anyway. That summer we travelled home where fresh and local ingredients were available, and I cannot tell you how much fresher our juices tasted! Even our young children commented on the heightened flavour and smell of their drink. That made me realise just how significant finding quality produce is, and I have tried very hard not to compromise since.*
> *(Anna, mother to children aged six and four)*

As you begin to practise eating in season, you will learn to appreciate the limited time spent with each fruit, vegetable, herb and spice. As the calendar changes, you will indulge in what is available, say goodbye to produce as its harvest comes to a close, and look forward to foods coming around again. I have to tell you that eating in this way gives you such an appreciation for food and how it was naturally made to taste.

Frozen Foods

Depending on where you reside, there may be times when you cannot find fresh, local or seasonal fruits and vegetables that your family likes. If this is your scenario, you might want to consider buying frozen. Frozen food is produce that is fresh at the time of freezing, and therefore maintains most, if not all of its nutritional value.

Please note that if you do decide to buy frozen foods for your family do take note of the use by date, and securely fasten the wrappings of produce you regularly open to use. Fruits and vegetables exposed to freezing conditions without adequate packaging are very likely to spoil.

Whole Grains

A whole grain is a grain that has kept all of its original parts. A whole grain food is complete as opposed to a refined food, which is not. It contains all of the vitamins, minerals, antioxidants and fibre that it was intended to have. Fibre will help to fill your child up for longer and maintain regular bowel movements.

Whole grain and whole wheat breads, pasta and rice, for example, is a healthier addition to your child's diet than white, processed foods, which to last longer have had much of the goodness taken out. Whole grain and whole wheat varieties of foods can be a wonderful addition to your family's diet.

Superfoods

In my opinion, all foods that promote health and provide life-enriching nutrients are super. For this reason, it is important to provide your family with a variety of produce to ensure they are getting all the goodness they need. The term superfood, given to those foods heralded as having increased nutritional value, if eaten alongside a healthy diet, can act as an important ally and furthermore help you to ward off illness, pain and even chronic disease. Noteworthy choices include beetroot, beans, berries, Greek yoghurt, green leafy vegetables, raw cacao, raw nuts and seeds, and wild salmon.

Quality Versus Quantity

When mothers begin to add more quality produce into the diets of their family I often hear concerns over the extra expense. Unfortunately, food is an unavoidable cost, so please be patient, because as you will begin to notice, there are areas where you will spend more and others where you will save. As already discussed, fresh, organic produce can be a little more expensive but the benefits, in my opinion, are more than worth it. Where you will save money, is having a shopping list and knowing exactly what it is you are buying before you hit the market or store, thus saving on items that are not necessary and will not be useful. That means buying only those foods in season, from local sources, for planned weekly recipes.

Keeping stock of what you have at home, in both your fridge and pantry, will also save you money. There is nothing worse than spending out on quality items only to realise that they have passed their expiration date. With fresh produce it is especially important to consume when ripe, so don't overbuy. A suggestion: doing a second weekly shop to buy fruits and vegetables might be sensible.

Bulk Buying

If you have the funds upfront (and the space to store) bulk buying quality produce will, over time, save you quite a bit of money, and is really very practical if you are consistently making the same types of foods for a large family. Bulk items that I typically buy include meat (that I can freeze), rice, flours, organic sugars, nuts, seeds and dates. Remember, if you do buy in bulk, to make a note of the use-by date and always store in the recommended way. For me, even though a lot of kitchen space is taken up I need less space for fresher items, which I am now purchasing on a more regular basis.

Something to Think About
The more you plan, prepare and cook at home, the more your family will begin to enjoy the benefits of eating more wholesome foods. This means you will buy fewer snack foods (that over time add up), and your family will likely eat out less (saving funds here also).

Strategies for Change:
- Eat and offer your family a balanced diet from a wide variety of local produce in season.
- Locate your nearest farm shop, market or nearby co-op; these locally run businesses offer a wide range of organic meats, fresh produce and home-made products. Many of them deliver right to your door.
- Consider a small vegetable patch or garden, or a simple herb box of your own. Some simple plants to try (in summer) include tomatoes and strawberries that grow quickly and in abundance

Positive Reinforcements

Every mother raising a child teaches desired behaviours and routines through repeated instruction and demonstration. Examples include brushing teeth morning and night to prevent cavities; regular washing of hands to promote good hygiene, and putting importance on rest periods and a strict sleep schedule to help foster good school and physical performance – the list goes on. We can do the same for nutrition and helping our child to eat well. Whatever is important to you as a parent predictably becomes important to your offspring. Children quickly adopt these routines as a way of life and over time not only understand the process but see the importance of it.

Make Every Morsel Matter

I have a personal rule when I am preparing or cooking food for my brood that no matter how small the snack or meal, every morsel on the plate should matter; that every ingredient, every item of food, every bite that they take should go in some way towards achieving optimal nourishment. It's not always easy, which is why meal planning, preparation, and a stocked kitchen go a long way towards assisting your success.

Start by adding an extra veggie, something raw at every meal, topping salads and grains with seeds and/or home-made dressings, include herbs and spices, powerful produce like ginger and beetroot to juices, add non-dairy milks to smoothies, etc. Your list and ambition to provide will soon become endless.

5 A Day

The 5 A Day movement was introduced by the World Health Organization (WHO), to promote the daily consumption of at least five portions of fruits and vegetables. For your family, this can be a good place to start adding in more fresh food, and will act as a reminder for the different types and amounts of produce one is expected to eat.

I carried out a similar project with my students when I asked them to bring a different fruit or vegetable in their lunch box for a week. We talked about the choices that were common to us and about other choices that were not. The children enjoyed learning about different fruits and vegetables, some of which, they had never seen or tasted before.

Rainbow

Offer, where possible, a colourful plate or bowl at every meal for your child. You will provide for him or her, a variety of whole produce that is rich in essential vitamins, minerals, phytonutrients and fibre, and successfully exceed the 5 A Day recommendation.

If one neglects to do this, a plate can be made very bland, unappealing to young eyes, and subsequently lacking in nutrient content. My boys, now accustomed to a colourful plate, are more eager to accept and enjoy what I prepare for them.

Sectioned Plate

Using a sectioned plate or imagining one, will further help you to add increased amounts and variation to your child's diet. Purchase or visualise a plate that has at least four sections; fill at least two of these with brightly coloured rainbow foods. Your child can help you to do this, and will probably enjoy doing so.

Something to Think About
When you provide your child with a diet full of nutrients, you leave very little room for him or her to experience hunger and cravings or the need to fill up on empty calories.

I don't always have complete control over my older children's food choices, especially as there are vending machines at school, but at home I try to encourage them, by us all eating healthy. I do this by making sure that the fresh produce we eat far outweighs the packaged.
(Leah, mother to children aged fourteen, thirteen, and twins aged five)

The Selection Process

By allowing your child to be very much a part of the process, choosing healthy foods together at the market or store will, over time, become enjoyable. My children, reluctant at first, now very much enjoy picking out their own choices. Let your child discover new produce, especially fruits and vegetables as they come in and out of season. Don't discourage them from varieties that you wouldn't normally buy (due to your tastes and preferences); let them take the time to choose for themselves. I had no idea that my oldest son liked mushrooms (because the rest of us did not) until he mentioned that he had eaten them at a friend's house and loved them.

Foods on Display

As your children begin to discover new foods, place chopped fruits and vegetables in containers towards the front of the fridge, where they can be taken. Additionally, provide fresh fruit in bowls, and nuts and seeds, and home-made goods in jars around your kitchen for everyone to see and help themselves to. Your children will have full access to these healthy choices when you are not around and if they are hungry.

Do remember to place age-appropriate and safe options for younger and smaller children but still within easy reach so they have the advantage of choosing healthy choices too. I have located cupboard space and one open shelf specifically for my two year old. I can't tell you how thrilled I am when I see him helping himself to an apple or asking me to peel a banana for him.

Just as your child will gravitate towards healthy produce that you leave out for them to see and access, less nutritious items will have the same appeal. If you have, let's say, leftover cake or other food from a birthday or event, put it away until you are ready (and willing) to offer it.

Remove and Replace

Without finding a replacement for the food you will remove, your family may begin to feel the effects of elimination and deprivation. This is certainly not something that I recommend for children. Despite the fact that your youngsters are unlikely to be eating or drinking a lot of the foods that cause withdrawal discomfort, say, from caffeine, for example, they may be somewhat reliant upon sugar and salt. These ingredients are regularly disguised in foods and it's labelling, but to make it easier for you please know that any packaged/processed foods (those that sit on a shop shelf for any period of time) will have some amount of preservative contained within them. Start by eliminating the more serious offenders from your cupboards and shelves as discussed in Chapter 1 and replace them with healthier alternatives, and even better, replace them with home-made varieties, that over time your family will like even more.

Focus more on foods you *can* eat rather than those you can't.

In the Kitchen

Even though I was not confident in the kitchen in the beginning I let Jul watch and help me out as much as possible. I wanted him and now his two brothers to see the effort and love that goes into making food for our family, but also I want them to be a part of all the processes as well. I know it can be tough when you may not have a lot of time to let your little ones assist you, but if you do you will see how much they love helping out and just how much they learn by doing so. I don't believe my children would have learned about using spices, the ways in which I make different milks, or the fun we have when making different varieties of muffins together, had I not included them. Now, my children will ask to make smoothies together, adding diverse ingredients to the mix each time, and I cherish watching them wait patiently for our home-made ice lollies to freeze so we can enjoy them with friends.

Appliances

To begin with (if you can), resist the temptation to go out and spend a lot of money on kitchen appliances that you may not need, or at least not yet. Concentrate firstly on getting a handle on some of the new foods that you and your family are now enjoying. Every mother's choice of how they will prepare food and the new techniques you will try, will be different, so be sure when you buy an appliance that you research fully, buy certified products, and decide on whether it is really something you will use for a long time to come.

When I first started this journey with my children I bought a simple juicer and a handheld blender. After a year I was certain that juicing was something that that we would continue to do every day and I spent money on a significant upgrade. Fast-forward more than five years and for all the additional foods I now prepare at home, I am the proud owner of a high-speed blender, a powerful food processor and a KitchenAid, most of which I use daily.

Picky Eaters

The subject of picky eating can be complex and for a number of reasons is commonly related to the emotional state of the individual child. With this in mind, I will refrain from delving too deeply into this topic. However, I confidently believe (because I have had a very picky eater of my own) that the practices I write about here and the support you show your growing child will go a long way towards preventing picky eating from occurring at all, or helping your child evolve out of it. With picky, fussy or stubborn eaters, it is even more important to get them involved. Grant them their independence and space by restraining yourself from having too much influence and control (see Chapter 5 for more detailed advice).

Please know that it takes a minimum number of times for your child to consume a food before they actually accept a taste or liking for it, so don't give up on those foods that you know are good for your child and their health requirements.

Rejection

If your child rejects a certain food, for example raw tomatoes, don't assume they won't like it in another form or within a recipe or meal – think pasta sauce. My youngest son won't eat avocado on its own, but will happily eat them mashed with bananas. My middle son doesn't like to eat oranges but loves fresh orange juice. For some children it is less about the taste and more about the consistency or texture – Jul refuses anything too mushy, so I offer him raw fruits and vegetables rather than the cooked, softer alternatives. It may take some time to work out what your young individuals' personal preferences are, but your investigations will be worth it.

After many months of Sahm refusing to eat raw veggies (because for him I have had to blend or cook them into a meal or snack), just a few weekends ago I noticed him happily helping himself to carrot sticks and dipping them into his tomato sauce! I hypothesised that this could be the solution for him: that he will indeed eat raw produce, but with something added. I have discovered since then that he prefers his apple with nut butter, cucumbers with goat's cheese and strawberries dusted with pure cacao powder (well, who wouldn't?!).

Snacking

From my observations, snacking is typically where mothers have the most difficult time sticking to their health routine. We are often out of the house, caught unawares by the timing of our child's hunger, or we are in a setting where other children are eating and offering our child food, and regularly end up scrambling for something to give them. Snacking should not be seen as an opportunity for you or your child to deter from nutrient-dense foods, but as a chance to include more.

Once you begin to recognise just how fundamental nutrition is, you fall in love with the desire to do anything and everything possible to feed your child well.

Packaged Foods

After a recent conversation with my girlfriends we realised that we had very different ideas about feeding our children snacks, which we concluded was down to us being raised in different parts of the world. While some of them thought of snacks as ready-made and packaged, as long as they were labelled as healthy, they would regularly feed them to their children. Others were raising their children similar to how they had been brought up on snacks that were only and always fresh, for example, fresh fruit, cut-up vegetables, home-breads, cereal bars and muffins etc., and the remainder of my friends didn't really believe in snacks or snacking at all, trusting that eating three to five nutritious and filling meals was enough to see their family through the day.

If you have become accustomed to giving your child food between meals, try if you can to cease relying too heavily on packaged foods. It used to be the case for me that I would buy more convenience foods, despite what I knew and the extra costs I incurred. Having lived away from my home country, with limited access to most of these foods, I soon learned to make my own.

Don't think for one moment that I was ever a dab hand in the kitchen either; I have had to teach myself everything. To be honest, it was never something I was interested in until I had to be. I found very quickly, however, that I grew fond of and accustomed to being able to offer my child something more wholesome, and for that reason, I have been highly motivated to continue.

Something to Think About
Filling up on snacks may hinder your child's accomplishments at mealtimes. Recommendations for growing children promote nutritious meals spread throughout the day. Therefore, refraining from too much snacking and letting your child build up a healthy appetite may work better for *your* child.

Strategies for Change:

- If you are switching to healthier types of foods (for example, from processed to whole grain/whole wheat varieties), start slowly – your child needs time to adjust to the new tastes and textures.
- Stay loyal to organic brands that you and your family like. Many starter companies competing against the corporate giants have a hard time staying in business, and your repeat custom is, therefore, encouraged.
- After a period of transition (this will be different for each family), stop buying and filling up your cupboards with produce that no longer suits your family's dietary needs. If it's not there, they can't eat it!

Be Prepared

I think you might agree that there has never been a better time to learn how to prepare food for your children. Making more of your family's food will allow you to actively monitor the individual choices of each child, ensure that they are all getting exactly what they need according to their age and activity levels, and enable you to feed them a range of foods that you know are life-giving.

Preparing more of your snacks and meals will admittedly take more time in the beginning. From my own viewpoint and from what other mothers tell me, being prepared means you suddenly become more effective, and in the long run, you spend fewer hours and less money even though the items on your shopping lists are now of a superior quality. You will feel much more dedicated to feeding your family well, and experience a real sense of achievement.

Something to Think About

The more prepared you are the less time you will waste, trying to rush meals together. When we are faced with a situation with little time and no supplies we can seriously compromise our efforts to do well. You will settle for food choices that are no longer part of the way you want to feed your family.

Prior Planning

If I plan ahead, I prepare the bulk of our family's foods at the weekend e.g. pasta sauces; curries; meat or meatless patties; soups; salad dressings; muffins; breads; date, seed and nut bars; and purees (for my youngest son). This way when I prepare dinner, for example (which is usually at our craziest time of day), I simply have to add quinoa, pasta, potatoes, rice, salad or vegetables, which let's admit, take very little time to prepare. And there you have it, a very healthy meal, very quickly.

> *Even though it takes time to prepare home-made foods and healthy snacks (lots of fresh fruits and veggies) for my family, it's really important to me. I do this to limit their desire for unhealthy foods that they may have access to.*
> *(Maryame, mother to children aged twelve, nine, five and three)*

Do it Yourself

Doesn't home-made food typically taste better? The flavour is superior and the fact that I know something was made by me or for me with care, attention and love makes me want it, and to share it, even more. For one, I know what ingredients went into making it, because I, or someone I trust, put them there.

Packaged foods, despite their persistence, can never quite live up to the quality of your home-prepared foods, because of the additives they have to include. So, it might take you a while to perfect your dishes, but isn't that half the fun? When your children see you preparing their food, food that they can partake in creating, that to me is worth the extra effort one hundredfold.

Home-made food becomes a part of your family. Your children will quickly recognise the tastes and smells that come from your kitchen, and the more foods you develop as your signatures dishes, the less you have to rely on store-bought foods and worrying about food labels and false health claims.

I will tell you once again that I am not a cook by any means, but that I have come to learn to love making some of my family's favourites. For me, being able to provide wholesome everyday items that I see my children enjoying means so much.

> *If a woman could see the sparks of light going forth from her fingertips when she is cooking, and the energy that goes into the food she handles, she would realize how much of herself she imbues into the meals that she prepares for her family and friends. It is one of the most important and least understood activities of life that the feelings that go into the preparation of food affect everyone who partakes of it. This activity should be unhurried, peaceful and happy because the energy that flows into that food impacts the energy of the receiver.*
> (Maha Cohan)

Healthy Alternatives

Now that you are thinking about or beginning to prepare the majority of your food at home, you may want to start with your family's favourites. The Internet and bookstores are awash with material describing in great detail what healthy ingredients you can use, where and how to find them, and the kitchen processes from start to finish. Now instead of completely removing foods that your family is familiar with, you are replacing them with something they recognise but with mounds of goodness and utter deliciousness! This strategy works particularly well with children who can show resistance to change.

Something to Think About

Avoid referring to your healthy home-made version of a food by the same name as its junk food equivalent. For example: in our home if I make healthy brownies, I call them *healthy* brownies. Some people may think this is counter-intuitive to their child then wanting the healthy version, but in my experience, if your child does not know that this food is good for them, they will easily select the unhealthy version (brownie) when it is offered outside of the home.

The Environment

I have spoken a great deal in this chapter about selecting produce that is local, seasonal and organic, all of which play a huge part not only in keeping your local environment and economy thriving, but in protecting our worldwide environment that we so urgently need to assist right now. Some more ways you can help in cutting back on inessential's and extra money, and ways in which to keep your produce fresher for longer, include:

Storing produce using glass containers. Just think: you might never need to buy foil, plastic wrap or plastic containers again. For all your storage needs (in or outside of the fridge and oven), glass jars, boxes and dishes are durable, maintain freshness and over time save you a lot of money. Glass containers also help to clearly display items, so that everyone knows where everything is.

BPA-free plastic might need to be used when glass containers are not appropriate, for example for your child's lunch box and drinks bottle. Some schools have a 'no glass' policy and so in these circumstances using BPA-free and refraining from the nasty chemicals found in many plastics is practical.

Stainless drinking straws are increasingly in popularity, I think due to more families making and drinking fresh juices and smoothies. They are environmentally friendly, easy to clean and can be used for a lifetime (we have had our batch for several years already). My own boys love really to use them.

Reusable food pouches that are BPA-free, recyclable, dishwasher- and freezer-safe and simple to fill and clean. Especially useful for parents and carers with young children, food pouches allow you to take more food on the go. I use these mostly for fruit and vegetable purees and smoothies, but they can be used for any food or meal that blends well.

You don't have to cook fancy or complicated masterpieces,
just good food from fresh ingredients.
(Julia Child)

Strategies for Change:

- Dedicate certain hours of the day or weekend to preparing foods.
- Store extra portions in the fridge or freezer for future use. (This is particularly helpful for days when you simply don't have any or enough time to prepare a nutritious meal from scratch.)
- Start creating a list of staple recipes that you will regularly make. Some of the easiest include fruit purees, hummus, jams, pasta sauces, muffins, muesli, non-dairy milks, nut butters, salad dressings, salsa etc.

Professional's Comments: Catherine Barnhoorn, Certified Integrative Nutrition Health Coach

As a recently celebrated author of the recipe book *Mila's Meals: The Beginning & The Basics* how important to you think it is for families to learn about the current food industry and how it affects what they eat and in turn, their health?

I think all parents are well aware of the importance and significance of nourishing their children. What I have come to realise though is that many parents mistakenly believe that the food industry is there to support them and help them in doing this. It is not. It is a business and its concern is primarily its bottom line – not the health and well-being of your child.

One only needs to read the ingredient labels of conventionally produced food products to understand this. Parents need to distinguish between filling their child's tummies, and nourishing their bodies. Real food nourishes a body – processed food simply fills it up. And then there is the whole matter of conventionally produced meat, dairy and fruits and vegetables and the GMO's, pesticides, growth hormones and antibiotics that are used in production – again, used not with the health of your child in mind. Food literally becomes the cells of your body. What you put in is what you are going to get out.

How vital is it for parents to prepare nutritious meals for their family?

When you prepare your own meals they are generally made from raw ingredients (real food) and therefore they are more nutritious than store-brought ready-made meals/food. But there is another nutrient in home-made food that is absent in all other pre-prepared food – Love. Cooking a meal from scratch is an act of self-care and self-love. It is making a statement that says I am worth this effort. There is so much that comes from a kitchen – besides a delicious and nutritious meal! Time in the kitchen is an act of love, for yourself and for your family. It is a time of connection – to the food and to each other. It is an opportunity to teach your children gratitude and respect – for food, and the earth and animals that provided it. If, as parents, our job is to create independent self-sufficient little beings that can confidently go into the world and shine their unique bright light, then teaching them how to nourish themselves and prepare their own (real) food is surely as important as any education we send them to school for.

You are raising your own daughter on a diet free from sugar (among other things), how beneficial do you believe this has been for her?

There have been benefits both for her – and I have to be honest and say for me too. Parenting is a big job, and a challenging one. It only makes sense not to make the job more difficult for you as a parent. Sugar affects child behaviour in so many ways – for example, it leads to hyperactivity (which I find difficult to deal with); tantrums and crankiness as the sugar-crash arrives; and, it over-excites children making getting them to sleep more difficult. In terms of physical health, the negative impact of sugar is vast. A child's immune system is still developing for the first few years of their life, which is why they are prone to getting the coughs and colds that go around. While this is a normal part of development, adding sugar to the mix means children are likely to get sick more often, and take longer to get better. As a parent, this means you are going to spend more of your time caring for your sick child.

My personal motivation to stick to the sugar-free way of eating is largely because there is Attention Deficit Disorder (ADD) in my daughter's gene pool. Sugar is known to trigger ADD and to worsen the symptoms. ADD is not something I want for her and I will go out of my way to prevent it.

My friends have often asked me how I can spend so much time in the kitchen, and time making all the free-from sweet food for Mila. For me it is a no-brainer. I would rather spend enjoyable time in the kitchen, than spending my time caring for a sick child, or disciplining an unruly one.

What advice can you offer those mothers who are struggling to raise healthy children in an overly processed environment?

Go natural/organic – with food as well as body-care and house cleaning products. Get back into nature at every opportunity. Where possible, grow your own food, or if you don't have the space to do that, shop at farmer's markets. Buy real food. Get back into the kitchen. Make real food. Make it with so much love, and so delicious that the processed, packaged food loses its appeal for your children. Know, in your heart, that by giving them the convenience food – you are not denying them! You are caring for them! Nourish their bodies, instead of simply feeding them.

What part do local farmers and growers and/or local businesses play in you providing the healthiest produce possible for your family?

I am blessed to live in a part of the world where there are many conscious food growers and farmers, and a couple of excellent markets where you can find all of your fresh produce. The town I live in is small, so there is a great sense of community and getting to know these food producers and farmer's is easy. It is amazing to be able to, for example, go to the goat farm and meet the goats and see first-hand how they are treated and nurtured and to know exactly where my goats milk comes from. As I now have complete mistrust of national food retailers, shopping at these farmer's markets or buying directly from the farmer has several benefits:

- I am getting organic, humanely raised, local produce.
- I know for a fact that it *really* is organic
- The produce is fresh, really fresh – like it has been picked that morning! So, it has not lost any of its nutritional value in transport or fridges.
- It is more cost effective than buying from a shop that will add a huge mark-up.

All of this and with the added feel-good factor that I am supporting small local businesses – enabling them to feed their families, instead of feeding a large national corporation's bottom line.

Food – Your Questions Answered

Can I still save money and feed my family quality foods?
I believe you can absolutely be budget-conscious and still feed your family well. Buying locally and seasonally will always be more cost-effective than buying foods shipped from overseas and out of season. Also, because you are now more health-aware you will find you endeavour to produce less waste. Meal planning can be another thrifty way of ensuring you only buy what you need and bulk buying is prudent.

I have heard great things about farmers' markets and shops but don't live close to any. Do I have any other options?
Many local farmers' markets and shops also deliver, or may be part of a wider co-op that can reach out to where you live. You can find out by looking online and doing a search for your area. Where my parents live in the England I have found one in particular to be reliable and their produce range outstanding. If I didn't have this resource I would find it hard to buy some of the locally produced organic and/or quality goods that I insist upon for my family.

My teenager watched an animal rights documentary and now wants to become vegan. Should I be concerned?
I think that it is admirable for a child of any age to be worried about the treatment of animals, especially those that will eventually become their food. It is quite normal for adolescents to experiment with different dietary regimes and so in this instance I would offer your support. From my professional point of view, as long as your child understands that they will need to replace foods that they are removing, I think that a vegetarian/vegan diet will actually promote more future health success than the current standard way of eating.

Chapter 3

FOCUS ON EDUCATION

Education is the most powerful weapon you have –

use it to change the world.

(Nelson Mandela)

Education is an effective tool if you are to steer your children towards better health. As a parent determined to help positively guide the next generation, getting the support you need in schools or being a capable role model is vital.

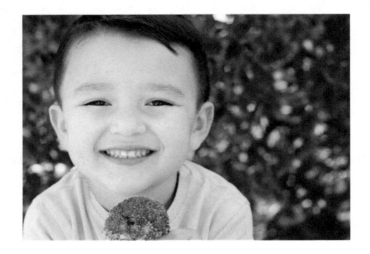

Health in the Classroom

As mothers, we cannot be expected to know it all or even pretend that we do. Perhaps you have reflected very little upon nutrition and educating yourself up to this point, but now that you have a family to take care of it's all that you can think about. The concept of health and everything that it incorporates is on-going and constantly changing. Even though this entire book is about empowering you as a mother to seek out and learn what you need to for the sake of your family's health, I do strongly believe that once your children are in a formal school setting, a school's co-operation is an essential component.

> *As a busy parent, I very much need the support of my son's school. With research gaining new evidence all of the time, it is important as parents to receive the on-going support and guidance we need for our children to remain healthy.*
> *(Nikki, mother to son aged six)*

As I have seen for myself in even the most brilliant of schools, teaching health, particularly nutrition and basic cooking skills, comes way down on a long list of subjects given priority in the classroom. Most schools have, in part, some sort of health programme built into their curriculum but it is often wildly out-dated, condensed over a one- to two-week period, and is led by the classroom teacher and not a certified health professional or health educator. Some schools even pick and choose what aspects of health will be taught, some concentrating only on wellness, others only on sports, some overlooking nutrition entirely. Other schools even have a bias towards one age group or another, focusing only on an early years programme and dropping it by secondary school, thus blocking students from taking their understanding further.

> *Health education is essential! I do worry, however, that they do not receive much in the way of an organised, up-to-date curriculum as one might expect or hope. If they did, I know this would benefit them greatly!*
> *(Kirsten, mother to children aged eleven and nine)*

Something to Think About

If your child's school does engage in certain health and nutrition practices these should be school-wide. What you can ask for, and hope to expect, is consistency.

Health Curriculum

In order for students to start thinking about food and what they are eating, to really understand what it means to be healthy, to prevent ill health, grow well, and to lead others by example, they need the implementation and support of an age-appropriate health curriculum carried out over the course of a whole school year. I feel strongly in saying that this should be given urgent priority.

Don't we already know that susceptibility to illness, learning and behavioural difficulties, lack of attention and tiredness are specifically related to limited health awareness and poor diet? So why aren't more schools more willing to make simple but effective school-wide changes that will provide an enhanced classroom environment, improved learning, and better behaviour?

Even at a very basic level, your child's school should be striving to teach awareness that:
- Health encompasses many factors (emotions, environment, nutrition, physical activity, sleep etc.).
- Regular practices and behaviours influence a person's overall health, positively or negatively.
- A healthy lifestyle can prevent illness and disease.
- It is important to seek up-to-date and regular health care (dentist, doctor etc.).
- Certain barriers can hinder personal and community health (access to modern healthcare, education, the environment, availability of foods, quality of foods etc.).
- Daily physical activity is significant in promoting overall wellness.
- There is a relationship between the food industry and its consumer.
- There is correlation between media and current technology and personal and community health.

(Source: Centers for Disease Control and Prevention (CDC).

Just as we hope a school's setting is broad enough to include the many individuals that attend, implementation of a health and wellness program should take into consideration multiple perspectives, cultures, religions and socio-economic status. A health curriculum needs to be inclusive. Health looks slightly different for different groups of people and this is something that we can all learn from (and be very excited about).

Wellness Policy

Whether your child's school has a wellness policy or not very much depends on where they go to school. If your child is fortunate the local schools authority will typically be responsible for implementing a wellness policy unique to the needs of each school, and insist upon a number of minimum requirements.

Schools with no wellness policy, but that are eager to promote better health, make no excuse for the limited resources they are equipped with and start making improvements on their own. By enforcing a wellness policy (regulated or not), that school is showing its staff, students and parents that health and its message are vital lessons that everyone deserves to learn. A wellness policy can be an exciting element of a school's curriculum, and can be amended to include new objectives and goals.

> *Having a food and health programme built into our school's curriculum has resulted in the majority of children (mine included), having an intrinsic awareness of what it means to be healthy. They are conscious of what is good for them and why other things are not, and even hold each other accountable for bringing healthy snack choices. Many parents (myself included) have been helped by their children to instil healthy habits at home as well. I am greatly appreciative of the school leadership for implementing a programme that creates a deeper awareness of healthy behaviours, and making it a part of the school culture.*
> *(Miss Selwaan, elementary principle and mother to six children)*

If your school's district or region does not enforce health and wellness lessons and food practices beyond what you see or expect, starting a dialogue with the school will be beneficial if you hope to advocate change.

Get Involved

The more you know about your child's school and what they offer, the better. Join the Parent Committee, and/or volunteer some of your time, no matter how little that may be. Ask about the wellness policy or about the health curriculum and other projects that the school may be promoting to increase health awareness. Just because the school doesn't have a specific agenda doesn't mean they are not actively pursuing ways to engage students in healthy learning and activities.

No matter how excited you are to start being more active, please don't be the type of parent who bulldozes in, expecting change immediately, because frankly that won't get you anywhere. Some schools are genuinely so overwhelmed with everything they have to do and comply with that they have sincerely neglected to see the health crisis and how they can be a huge catalyst for change.

Setting the Scene

I really don't believe I thought much about or appreciated the classroom environment until I began to teach in a school myself. When you impart information in such a setting you set the stage for learning to take place. A classroom's conditions are set up to facilitate the teacher-to-student connection, thus enabling the teacher to engage with his or her students to successfully teach, hand over knowledge and demonstrate vital skills. When your child has the privilege of receiving health and nutrition classes on a regular basis at school, like any other subject, they will become aware of its inclusion and importance.

> *Obviously, the classroom is a great place to receive health information.*
> *(Laura, middle school teacher)*

Student-to-student participation is also vital and is not something you can easily replicate at home. Among their peers, children tend to cooperate better, stay stimulated for longer, show greater signs of motivation and effectively help one another to learn more. What better environment is there, then, to teach the fundamentals of nutrition than school?

Teachers Learning Health

If all teachers could be taught the fundamentals of health and nutrition, they too could promote healthy practices in their own classrooms (this can be done by offering a handful of basic workshops or seminars). From my experience, teachers are extremely open to this type of encouragement and instruction. Teachers are busy people, focusing for the most part on one subject or one age group, which takes up a considerable amount of their time and energy. They may not be informed on current health or nutrition guidelines, or the practices that they can use to promote health in the classroom, which in turn benefits their students to learn, socialise and behave better.

From what I have witnessed, teachers are more than happy to take on a standard set of guidelines that will further their students' learning and development. When a school takes the time to do this, you see some excellent ideas being put into place. Teachers, encouraging students to drink more water, practising good hygiene through role play, creating an incentive programme among peers to motivate children to bring healthier snack and lunch choices, inspiring students (of all ages) to cook, and making birthdays and other celebrations about the child and not about the food.

Why Lessons Alone Are Not Enough

Possibly the thing I love most about teaching is being witness to the remarkably fast and surprisingly positive response that children of all ages have when learning about the importance of the food they eat – after all, it is something that they do day in, day out. Yet, as any good teacher will tell you, learning alone isn't enough. A student needs to study consistently, put the subject into practical use in everyday situations and understand and connect with that subject before they really master it.

I think the concept of health is very important. I believe it's equally as important as learning maths, reading and writing. Children develop habits, likes and dislikes at a very young age, and for this reason, it's important to incorporate health into the everyday programme.
(Jenny, elementary school principle)

My personal role and experience within a school have shown me that definitely, lessons alone (particularly when they are condensed over a short period) are not enough. They are most certainly a start, but we owe our children much more than this. Having a weekly period dedicated to health and nutrition allows the student to learn continuously (as they do with other subjects), and do more than simply learn from a book. Giving more time to health allows the student to participate in practical activities such as food tasting, basic cooking skills, tending to a small garden or vegetable patch and more.

It was my intention from the outset to include health and nutrition education as a fundamental part of our school system. Providing school lunches as part of the health programme, I knew, was very important for our students, and after asking myself how to go about this correctly, I recruited Tamar and a kitchen full of staff. Six years later we continue to make seasonal, organic, age-appropriate hot lunches for over two hundred students. The health class that the children partake in reinforces the health benefits of what they are eating in the cafeteria, and provides them with the knowledge

to make their own well-informed choices. I very much believe that the mind and body work hand in hand, and when children learn from an early age how important health and its practices are, they continue with this for life. This, I am certain, is one of the most important skills we can teach our children."
(Aida Adnan, elementary school founder and director, and mother to five children)

You may be wondering if this is conceivable for your child. I have had the greatest good fortune to work at a school that, through a lot of hard work and passion, has made this happen.
It is desperately needed and entirely possible for all schools.

School Food

All over the world (especially in the past few years), a great many schools, having discovered the importance of nutritious food for students, have significantly upgraded their school lunch menus. On a recent trip to visit to a number of primary schools in the UK I was pleased to see that producing healthy meals had become a priority to which the schools were happily adhering. Using more local suppliers and even taking some of the food from their own schools gardens and greenhouses, providing a number of nutritious, age-appropriate options including vegetarian and special meals to meet other dietary requirements, it seemed to me that the children were enjoying school lunches at their very best.

With a strong correlation between diet and academic performance, school meals can be a great educational support. Nutrient-dense, hot meals have been praised time and time again for their inclusion in schools. In many parts of the world, children rely on school meals (sometimes free) as the most wholesome and reliable meal of their day.

Something to Think About
Adequate school meals not only support the children who are eating them, but also us as their parents. What mother has not had the dilemma of what to pack for school lunches, assuming all the ingredients you need are consistently stocked at home? (I know I have!) When substantial meals are provided at school, that's one nutritious meal a day taken care of.

Eating in the Cafeteria

Children who partake in a school's food system can benefit greatly from the influence of others. If the environment is supportive and all children are eating the same nutritious foods, we see positive peer pressure to conform to healthier habits, such as trying new foods and good table manners. Children really begin to look forward to their lunch, and not just because they are hungry. Therefore, if you do have the option of enrolling your child in a nutritious school lunch programme, I would encourage you to jump at the chance!

Unfortunately, this will not be the standard in every school. Try not to have too much anxiety over it, but offer to work with your school to provide them with information and suggestions to generate change.

> *At the beginning of the school year, only two of my students would try vegetables or salad while eating lunch in the school cafeteria. Now seven months later, with on-going health lessons in the classroom and teacher-student support in the cafeteria, all but a few of the children happily eat the majority of foods that are on their plates.*
> *(Rhonda, elementary teacher)*

Students Choosing Menus

When I first began to implement the menus in a school, I didn't think about the many cultures we were serving or asking for the input from parents and students. Just one month in I realized that although the meals were indeed nutritious, they were not familiar to some of the children. From that experience and many years on I regularly ask the students for their ideas (which they enthusiastically love to give), and modify the menus to include seasonal foods and traditional recipes.

> *I think one of the greatest assets of the health programme is allowing kids the input to think about what foods they like and the empowerment they feel when they are asked for their involvement. Once they realise they will be heard, and that their opinions matter, they start to care about the food they will be eating and begin to create healthy recipes within the guidelines that they are also learning in health class. It can be hard to make a nine- or ten-year old care about veggies, but when they get to think about how they will present these foods, suddenly healthy foods don't seem so bad. They love being involved in the process and seeing the end results. As I write this, my own class are anxious to see next month's menu and the contributions they have made.*
> *(Beth, fourth- and fifth-grade teacher)*

Home-Brought Food

I am asked time and time again for suggestions for a healthy snack or lunch box. If your child's school does not provide adequate on-campus meals then providing your child with an assortment of foods that will sufficiently fill him or her up is essential.

Just as consistent, nutritious foods are important for a school to provide, so are the guidelines that I would like schools to put in place for parents as well. Having a set of standards, ideas and suggestions for snack and lunch box choices that parents can look to for guidance is a huge support for mothers. This is another area where the school can provide information via the school handbook, online resources or workshops (which are particularly valuable). When students see other students eating the same or similar foods to them, the healthy encouragement and cycle continues; it's positively profound to watch.

> *I love watching the students inspecting each other's foods knowledgeably informing each other that this food or that is good for the body and how, and saying things like 'Actually, water is the best drink for you!' And I'm thinking to myself how amazing it is that these kids have learned so much without really knowing it, I mean, they are actually reading the box labels! This is huge! And I know if they are talking about it at school, they are certainly talking about it at home.*
> *(Sara, third-grade teacher)*

Please Note

No child should be made to feel singled out or excluded for not having the 'right' foods in their lunch box. By offering parents guidelines, lists of available food items and above all the school's support, one can hope to expect for more appropriate food choices, but if this is not the case the child should not be made to suffer. The school and its supporting staff are there to help both the child and parent in this circumstance.

Junk Foods on the Premises

This is a catastrophe for so many reasons. Retailers being allowed to sell junk or fast food in or close to schools is directly undermining children's right to health and their on-going education. Think of the vision and all the hard work that goes into the implementation of a school's health and food programme (no matter how small it may be), and the lack of integrity this demonstrates.

Schools would never invest time, energy and hours of teacher's training into, say, a maths curriculum for them to later decide on an unsuitable, below-par programme that yields less than desirable results for their students. The thing to ponder here is why individual schools have the power to choose to sell produce on the behalf of fast food outlets and junk food options in the first place? As a health professional working in a school, I realise the bravery (not to mention the additional time and effort) it takes any administration to go above and beyond what is expected of a school and this should be commended.

Why, then, contradict that good work through the blatant exposure to non-nutritious, convenience food and drinks that so clearly undermine all the good being done? What really stunned me to learn is that in some schools, while foods prepared and sold by the school need to meet specific nutritional guidelines, foods from other outlets, including soft drinks, chocolate bars and other nutritionally low options, are allowed! As you might have guessed, the answer again is down to money. Schools believe that they can make more money in this way rather than by running their own food services.

Food Rewards

Using food as a reward in the classroom is a concept I find hard to understand, primarily because it is not conducive to the learning environment, not to mention undermining the health curriculum being taught. Teachers know that rewards are an extremely effective way of encouraging positive behaviours, however, the most effective rewards should not be food- or material-based but those that are favourable to the overall mission of the school. Rewards involving recognition for good actions, privileges and other opportunities for development are more persuasive ways to help students in the classroom.

Something to Think About

With little exception the offered food rewards are almost always nutritionally poor. Another issue to consider is, that unless you enquire, or your child tells you, you may not even know that foods are being given in the classroom! If you are a mother, like me, who puts effort into making quality, healthy snacks and lunch boxes, you might really loathe to seeing half of it come home because your child has filled up with junk foods that have been unnecessarily handed out during class time.

In Praise of Teachers

And so this is why it's imperative for a school's administration to support and educate its teachers on health and provide clear guidelines for the classroom, and I do believe this is one area that is positively being addressed. So, it is hats off to all the remarkably brilliant teachers out there who are in in step with their students, who know all too well the signs of disruption caused by poor food choices, and who refrain from giving such rewards.

It is also worth mentioning that with a growing number of children with food allergies it is now considered unsafe to offer foods that may not be suitable for all. It is also unfair to exclude these students from activities involving unsuitable food rewards solely because they are not permitted to eat them.

Celebrating Health

At school, children celebrate all sorts of achievements. Teachers praise students for their reading and writing ability, and at times throughout the year parties or other celebrations are given to reward the whole class for good behaviour or other academic successes. Celebrating health brings honour to a subject that is imperative to the lives of each and every one of us, and allowing students the opportunity to reflect on the many aspects they have learned thus far will acknowledge this. Observing the internationally recognised days of health week is just one fun way to respect the importance of the health and wellness curriculum. Students of all ages can bring in healthy foods to share, nutritious juices and smoothies can be made at school and given out to try, parents can be invited to join their children at lunch, games with a host of physical activities can be organised, and even money can be raised through donations or other planned events in recognition of a chosen health charity.

Student Teaches Parent

It is very often the case that once a child begins to love a subject, they bring home and share what they are learning. The theme of nutrition is particularly appealing to a young child, especially if the practical opportunities have been put in place for the child to experience. Sharing these skills with the people they love brings great joy to the young child, and something of so much importance must be nurtured. This precise situation provides you as a parent with a brilliant opportunity to expand on a topic that your child has shown interest in. Ask more questions, seek to find out what they know already and develop their understanding, share ideas and offer further encouragement.

I really like it when we make healthy juices and smoothies in health class. I have learned to make them at home now and can share them with my mum, dad and sisters.
(Student, aged six)

Strategies for Change:

- If you have concerns about any aspect of the current health curriculum or practices at your child's school, speak to the appropriate person(s). How can a school work better at providing for its students if they don't hear otherwise?
- Get involved. No matter how small your contribution, you can be a valid part of the school's community.
- Show enthusiasm for your child's learning by asking questions and showing support. If there is a particular topic that he or she has shown interest in, follow it up at home.

At Home Educator

If there wasn't enough for mothers to do already, the new task of being the at-home health educator may at first seem daunting, but let me reassure you, it is actually quite fun and let's not forget, undeniably valuable. Until I began to teach I was not really conscious of the enormous part I could play in the health education of my own children. When I saw the overwhelmingly positive response from students in the classroom, I changed my mind, and knew I could indeed do something similar at home. Now, without it seeming like just another homework task, I subtly reinforce what they are learning in the classroom and guide my children to talk about and practise healthy habits as often as I can.

There are some really remarkable books and online resources that offer a great way to start health conversations at home, and let's not forget everyday practices like food shopping, food preparation and cooking to help get your family involved and talking. In fact, you don't really have to see it as being a teacher to your children at all, but as finding the 'healthy' *in* the things you do at home and passing this along. The idea is, if you can find a way to promote being healthy among your child's everyday activities, you will be guaranteed that your child will become more responsive to health expectations and strive to make healthier choices as they go about their day.

Personally, I feel that home is one of the best places to learn about health, where it can be modelled and reinforced.
(Laura, mother to children aged fifteen and thirteen)

Something to Think About

As you begin interpreting the guidelines offered to you, and as you and your family start to put habits into place, pat yourselves on the back from time to time. Putting in so much effort to something that will be truly transforming deserves acknowledgement and praise.

Eating for Nutrient Content

As an educator, I cannot emphasise enough how essential it is to find a way to make your children understand how crucial it is to eat with nutrition in mind. Many of the tips and tricks suggested throughout these chapters will encourage your child to eat better, and yet a simple age-appropriate explanation and encouragement that you can reiterate over and over will help them truly understand and aid your efforts much further.

Role Play

In the classroom, for younger children, I explain how the body is like a flower that needs the sun, air, water, food and shelter to grow tall and strong. I explain that without these components the flower can become sick and lifeless. I ask them what food the flower eats and we talk about all the nutrients in the soil that the flower gets, and how for us that is like fresh produce full of vital vitamins and minerals. I ask them if the flower needs doughnuts, or soda or sweets, of course they say no, and so I ask them if *they* need doughnuts, or soda or sweets. They laugh, and give a resounding no in response. Having a picture or actual plant or flower in your home will act as a good reminder.

For older children we talk more candidly, reinforcing why good nutrition from real foods is important. We learn how foods play an essential role in the engineering of their bodies, and alternatively what processed, food-like substances and chemicals do and the disruptions they cause. When a child truly comprehends this, they start to think about nutrition in a whole new light. They understand that although they might like the taste of sweets, for example, it is because of the high sugar content and not because the body actually needs or wants it. They begin to learn that instead of providing something for the body, this food and others like it are actually taking something away. When I see this realisation in my students, and the impact it has on their food choices, I am filled with confidence knowing they are growing up to be positive health advocates, not only for themselves but for those around them. What a great start this can be for our next generation.

> *The most valuable thing I think I have learned so far is understanding what I really need to eat and what I don't.*
> *(Student, aged ten)*

Trust Your Intuition

If you are a new parent, or new to the different health concepts mentioned here, and would simply like to add in more health practices then the remaining chapters in NOURISH will help you to do that. Remember also that you don't have to be a teacher to teach – your personal relationship with your child or children and the experiences you have together, will mean you will know what it is that they need and when.

> *When Flynn was a baby I looked for the answers to so many questions I was asking, but couldn't always find them. So I just started using intuition and how I was raised. My mother was a stay-at-home mother and had strong opinions about healthy food – it's not like she imparted her advice or even that I asked for it, but obviously it was something that was just taught. I think it's mostly common sense that I use for my child now, and having fun with each other.*
> *(Emily, mother to son aged three)*

What I would like to say, if I may, is do try to have fun with your family's learning! It will make the role of an at-home educator so much easier for you, and much more enjoyable for your children!

Strategies for Change:
- Add colourful, fun and applicable books that feature actions or stories of positive health practices to your child's bookshelf. Your child will inevitably pick them up and will enjoy reading them with you.
- If there is a health practice that you are new to, information you have yet to learn or have a new recipe to try out, do it alongside your child. Showing your child that you are learning something new with them will encourage them and show them how important doing something towards better health is.
- Get everyone involved. Include members of your entire family to help you reinforce learning at home. For example, if my husband hears me telling my child why a particular food is good for him, he will bring it up another time with a book or in conversation.

Your Support Network

Feeling inspired? Stay motivated by reaching out and finding support.

Professional Support

In my occupation as a health counsellor, I typically work with families for a period of six weeks or more. It is utterly rewarding as one, two or all members of that family begin to see health for the glorious gift that it is. Through support, education and at-home practice, families start to take seriously the issue of nutrition, and depending on the age of those included, will hold themselves responsible and maintain new habits.

> *Working with a health professional really changed my life for the better. In a relatively short period of time, I learned how to make better choices. I thank Tamar for starting my healthy eating revolution that has led to the whole family being healthier.*
> *(Hala, client)*

If you are finding it difficult to get started or need help with specific issues related to the health of your family, seeking professional support could be of great assistance. It's not that you can't or won't succeed on your own, but being accountable to someone else can really set you off in a positive direction. If you can't or don't want to spend money on a health professional, maybe someone you know has experience with a particular health area you are interested in and you could trade services?

> *Learning with Tamar changed our lives in terms of the nutrition knowledge we acquired. The habits we learned have given us the ability to raise our children healthily. Tamar was so professional, caring, current, and well researched in her approach. We cannot thank her enough for what we've gained.*
> *(Meryn and Dean, clients and parents to twins aged one)*

Like-Minded Others

For me, my personal journey as a mother has been delightfully enriching and strongly supported by the involvement of like-minded others. There is nothing better than sharing stories, offloading worries or seeking advice with another mum (or a group of them) who is going through much the same as you, as we all know motherhood can be difficult. With so much information available to interpret, particularly when your time is suddenly limited (and precious), having friends for support is crucial.

> *For health support I reach out to like-minded families.*
> *(Andrew, father to son aged ten)*

As much as it is important to share your parenting experiences with others, do focus on finding those who genuinely support you. You may have a huge friend base but choosing those that will enhance your parenting journey and experiences rather than invalidate them, will benefit you more. Expect that everyone will have their opinion, that's fine, and one should respect that, but having someone inflict those opinions on you is something else. Those people who truly value your friendship and your role as a mother will know the difficulties and hardships that come with it, and only want to embrace times spent together, good and bad.

Online Resources

As long as you are able to sift through the unnecessary and pick out the relevant material for you, online resources can offer a huge wealth of information. When you do find a particular source that you trust, whether it is an organisation or individual offering advice, I recommend staying loyal to them (at the most, a few). A really good health expert (professional or self-taught) will pack their websites, bringing you up-to-date information because they really care about getting their health message across. In all my years devoted to health issues, and despite the hundreds of books I have read on related issues I only subscribe to a handful of online contributors (see Resources and Recommendations). My reasons for this are as follows:

- I love getting to know the expert and how he or she relates to me, and my particular health journey.
- I really don't have the time to spend on additional research.
- Because spending insurmountable hours trawling the Internet will likely only

succeed in confusing and contradictive messages, leaving me more clueless than when I began.

Building a network of like-minded people is essential, and by asking, exploring and reading on-line, you can find almost everything you might be looking to learn.
(Leigh-Jane, mother to daughters aged eight and five)

Books

I adore books and think they are a wonderful addition to anyone's home library. I believe that it is more peaceful to sit down with a book than to search the Internet, but just like I warned you when doing your online research, knowing which book to pick can be difficult. I consider the best books to be those passed on or highly recommended by others. Please note that books pertaining to health, specifically those with a scientific base, will inevitably need updating. Books that act as a guide, like NOURISH will offer you information at a moment's notice, and dipping in and out of their pages as you need to will serve you well. Recipe and cookbooks are always enticing, but do if you can do take a quick look through them first. I cannot tell you how many such books I have gathering dust on my shelves that on closer inspection are not really suited to my family's needs. Either that or the ingredients are difficult or impossible to obtain, or simply not agreeable to our tastes.

Strategies for Change:
- Basic nutrition education is the key to getting started. Try not to feel overwhelmed by the amount of information on offer. Use your judgement, and seek out those professional and non-professional sources that you feel most comfortable with.
- Share insightful and supportive information or people of interest with others. Having solid recommendations for doctors, carers, books and other must-have-resources, saves so much time money *and* effort.
- Trust your mother's intuition, it will serve you well.

It is not what you do for your children but what you have taught them to do for themselves that will make them successful human beings.
(Ann Landers)

Professional Comments:
Katee Inghram, Classroom Teacher, Language Co-ordinator and Coach.

As a classroom teacher what has your experience been with encouraging healthy practices?

My students enjoy learning about different ways to stay healthy. We talk about taking care of our minds and our bodies in order to be really, holistically happy. When we have been sitting for a while, we take brain breaks and use movement to refocus. At times, we do yoga after lunch or during transitions. Sometimes we lie on the floor and participate in guided meditation. These practices, in addition to following through with the school's expectations for healthy eating, help our classroom community identify as growing, healthy human beings.

Do you think teachers are comfortable teaching a health and wellness curriculum?

As with any curriculum, it's important for teachers to feel they have adequate prior experience or the amount of training they need with the material they are expected to teach on the topic. Because individual teachers' experiences vary so greatly, I think it's important for a school organisation to outline its vision for health and wellness and share that with teachers school-wide to ensure consistency in content and delivery and a clear progression in student learning.

How important do you think it is for teachers to show healthy practices in the classroom (e.g. making nutritious food choices and refraining from consuming unhealthy foods or drinks)?

It's critical for teachers to model healthy choices. Students are keenly observant and actions are so much more powerful than words. Teachers are teaching, and messages are sent and received all of the time! Students are constantly noting what a teacher says and does. In simple ways, a teacher can share a healthy lifestyle with his or her students. For example, it's good for the students to hear about what time you go to sleep, when you make a point to relax, and what you do to stay active. It's helpful for children to see teachers set goals and get excited about something that benefits their well-being. This kind of powerful teaching is not done with a health unit and never talked about again, instead, it's a casual, rolling conversation that comes back around when it's appropriate for sharing. Frequent, authentic mention of healthy choices allows students to see that health is a true priority and a way of life.

Many schools don't have a formal, organised or up-to-date health curriculum. What are your thoughts on this?

A formal, organised health curriculum is necessary in schools today. Having a set curriculum for health and wellness places the topic as a priority and is one way to ensure the defined standard is being met.

As a mother to two young children what are your hopes for their future in terms of health education in their remaining years at school? What can you do to assist this?

I hope that my children are provided with the opportunity to spend time talking about health and wellness with their peers. I would like my boys to be exposed to the decisions others are making and then decide what they feel is right and best supports their own well-being. I hope my children are supported in a holistic manner, and that they can learn more about nutrition, fitness, relaxation, lifestyle etc. As a parent, I can model, support and encourage choices that nourish my child and hope that because I am just one influence, other influences are doing the same.

Education – Your Questions Answered

The information my children are receiving in health class is noticeably out of date – what can I do about it?

Firstly, the fact that your children are having health lessons is great but I agree with you that if the lessons are not up to date and current with our world at large then they might be being taught the wrong message. I don't believe that this is the school's objective; I just think that expectations in this subject area are low, and unless something is done to bring about change, then they are very likely to continue with the same expired programme. What you can do as a concerned parent is voice your point of view with the administration, the schools board and/or at the parent-teacher committee meetings. It is very likely that others share your opinion and want change too. You might be surprised to find that when a number of well-intentioned parents voice their support for improvement, the school works with them to provide this.

A home-made item from my son's lunch box was removed by his teacher and he was told it was not healthy? Is this a practice that schools are applying now? Is this considered acceptable?

This is one area that needs to be approached with great caution and care. Not all parents and guardians have the funds to budget for high-quality health foods or organic brands and more commonly some don't know what to look for (and I don't blame them because it's difficult). I very much understand a school's need to prohibit the obvious unhealthy culprits – soft drinks, sugar-laden juices and milks, crisps, fried foods, and of course chocolate bars and sweets – but when a school bans or begins to 'police' food (by taking it away without replacing it with a healthy alternative) they can find themselves in somewhat tricky territory. I think what the school should do first is to write a short letter or email to you as the parent, giving you the opportunity to explain your choices or the home-made varieties you have made. I feel that if a school is doing all they honestly can to support health, then both the parent and child will make choices that are indeed nutritious and accepted, and it is then in the best interests of the everyone to trust that what's in the child's lunch box is right for them. No child, especially at such a young age, should be made to feel awkward (or hungry) within the classroom setting for food that has been packed from home.

At my daughter's school they have been told not to bring in a cake or foods for birthday celebrations. Am I justified in feeling sad that this is no longer acceptable?
Sharing foods brought in from home or from outside caterers is generally considered unsafe due to those who might suffer from food allergies. Sharing birthday cake with friends is of course a special event but one that I feel strongly should be done outside of the classroom. If your child's school does have a wellness policy the offering of birthday cake (which, let's be honest, generally contains a vast amount of brightly coloured frosting) will be in direct conflict with its guidelines. That is not to say that celebrating your child on their special day is not important. At my children's school they get to choose how they would like to be honoured – with a song, a picture, a special hat etc. For all children celebrating in this way, not having a cake is of little significance and one that they quickly forget.

Chapter 4
FOCUS ON HEALTH

My mission in life is not to merely survive, but to thrive.

(Maya Angelou)

Is human health simply the freedom from illness or injury? According to the World Health Organisation it is *the complete physical, mental and social well-being of a person and not merely the absence of disease or infirmity.*

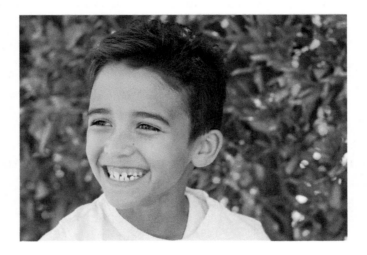

Holistic Health

All areas of a life worth living need attention, devotion and care, and health is certainly a precious gift worth working for. To attain and maintain health, I believe, means to pay close attention to and wholeheartedly seek out wellness in all areas of one's life, all of the time. One aspect does not, and cannot, work well on its own; we are indeed a sum of our parts.

Your child's longevity is very much in your hands. Providing holistic health care is helping him or her to live their life to the fullest. When you raise your child with both the bigger picture and the whole picture in mind, you are very much aware that what you do now for your child will affect their health and well-being in the future.

Experiencing Ill Health

Jul's health experiences meant that my husband and I would internally agonise and constantly worry over the prospect of something happening to him (or our other boys) again. At the very same time those experiences made us realise that you can never take health for granted and no matter what position you may find yourself in, taking the steps towards whole health awareness through self-education, advocacy, prevention, practice and your role as the at home-educator will bring you the most success, and also a calmer state of mind.

A Different Approach

Years ago it was commonplace to expect or even demand a prescription upon visiting the doctor. Without this, people felt the physician was suspicious of the symptoms they were complaining of. Hearing that your child has a diagnosed illness, and is being given the drugs to fight it, provides parents with the assurance that they can assist their child to better health. Medicines, however, are not always necessary. Knowing that any drug we take is used by the body as a whole, and not just in the one particular area where it's required, may lead you to seek alternatives.

I hold doctors' opinions in high regard and know that quality drugs have an essential part to play in the recovery from many illnesses, yet it is important to understand that there is virtually no known drug that does not have any side effects. I am always inspired, therefore, when my child's paediatrician looks to me for clues regarding my child's current ailment, when and how it started, on-going symptoms and so on. I am further encouraged when he suggests alternative treatments that may not only eradicate symptoms of the malady at this stage, but act as a powerful preventative against future illness.

Please hear me when I say that I emphasise wholeheartedly with the somewhat scary decision to take a less-than-traditional route when it comes to treating a sick child. If you are from the Western world as I am, drugs have become commonplace, sadly. Something easy to obtain and even easier to administer. Having spent time in different countries with people from different backgrounds, I have come to place huge value on alternative methods. Such treatments place less stress on the body and allow the system to manage its pain and healing more naturally.

> *Living abroad, I miss many of the things about my home country. Where I come from it is not at all common to give your children antibiotics – rather, we are encouraged to help our children manage their symptoms, let the immune system do its job, and allow the body to heal naturally. Of course medicines are sometimes required and will be taken, but they are not the first things mothers think about or use. I listen daily to a local radio station from where I grew up and am reminded of this practice by government advertisements that warn against the overuse of antibiotics and the effects on the growing child. I feel so lucky to have been raised in an environment that promotes health, and even though I am now raising my own children somewhere less familiar I can still model and insist on those practices from home.*
> *(Vera, mother to children aged seven and five)*

Something to Think About

Even with no treatment at all, a large number of basic illnesses will remedy themselves, if the body is given adequate time and the rest it needs.

Complementary and Alternative Medicines (CAM)

Complementary and alternative medicines and therapies have never been so popular. Commonly used by those seeking an alternative to over-the-counter treatments, they can be an excellent consideration for your family. CAM medicines and therapies are typically non-invasive and work to stimulate the body's natural healing response. Many integrative doctors (as well as some mainstream ones) support CAM therapies, promoting the part they play in a greater mind-body connection. Such doctors will regularly prescribe them alone or in combination with conventional drugs and methods. Alternative therapies that you might like to learn more about include homeopathy, home-made remedies, massage, certain forms of exercise and changes to an existing diet.

> *I am a strong believer in steering away from modern chemically-based medicines as much as possible and have made the choice to treat my family via more natural alternatives such as homeopathy, traditional Chinese medicine and energy healing. (Fifi, mother to children aged nine and seven)*

Tried and Tested At-Home Formulas (That Work)

Whether your child has a runny nose or cold, a stomach upset, low fever or mosquito bite, simple home remedies can offer fast and comforting relief.

Bumps, Bruises and Bangs
I started using homeopathy from the time Jul was born and since then it has played a big part in the lives of our entire family. Arnica, which is probably the most common remedy, found in pillule, cream or gel form, is a wonderful remedy for any type of contusion (except those that have opened the skin). Give a pillule orally or apply cream or gel immediately and at regular intervals after your child's fall.

Runny Noses or Colds
At the first sign of sniffles and sneezes, think about starting a nasal rinse on a regular basis. Add a tiny amount of sea salt to a cup of warm (previously boiled) water, and simply have your child sniff up some of the solution from your hand or theirs, blocking each nostril in turn as they do so. After each nostril has been rinsed have your child blow their nose.

Stuffy Noses
I add a little sesame or olive oil (using a cotton bud) to my children's noses every night before bed. This prevents their noses from becoming dry due to hot or arid weather conditions during the warmer months, and avoids stuffiness caused by central heating during the colder months.

Sore Throats

The beginnings of a sore throat can quickly grow into an infection at a young age, so relieving this symptom and hopefully its cause will benefit your child enormously. Once again, using a solution of a small amount of sea salt in a cup of warm (previously boiled) water and gargling regularly will help. If your child will tolerate drinking warm water or warm herbal teas, this will remove some of the pain too.

Coughs or Sore Chests

A cough is the body's natural way of expelling irritants from the throat and airways, and therefore over-the-counter cough mixtures that suppress the cough will only add to your child's discomfort and illness in the long run. A cough can be extremely irritating, not to mention keeping your child from sleeping at night, and at times may be a symptom of croup or asthma. As a mother it is important to monitor your child's cough and breathing for any signs of change. One remedy that I have used for all my children is golden honey paste.

Golden Honey Paste (Good for children, as the taste is sweet!)
Ingredients
1/4 cup organic turmeric powder
1 cup high-quality manuka honey (can be found in some supermarkets, health food stores and online).
To Make
Simply stir the turmeric powder and manuka honey together until completely blended. Store in an airtight jar, away from sunlight, and use within two weeks.
Dosage
Begin to offer your child golden honey paste as the cold season approaches (this will be different depending on where you live in the world), one teaspoon morning and night (more if your child is already complaining of symptoms).

Please note that honey is not recommended for children under one year.

The Immune System

Your child is very likely to get sick at some point and experience symptoms of discomfort and unease, but what we all hope for is that our child only endures what is naturally expected. As much as we detest ill health, it is a normal and essential process, required to build a strong immune system. If you understand that the immune system is the body's greatest form of protection, you might then appreciate the importance of taking care of it.

Nutrition plays a huge part in the developmental stages and on-going maintenance of the immune system, not forgetting the vital role it also plays in the restoration process when the body is under attack or weakened from illness. If you research and look, you will find numerous ways in which to boost your child's immune system when they are ill or recovering from sickness. What I hope to shed more light on is the huge importance of building a solid foundation from the start, and developing it further from there.

A healthy immune system is like a strong foundation for a house. Your little one's immune system is developing from the time they are born and for the next seven years of their lives – and then that is the one that has to see them through for the rest of their lives. I believe it is our duty as mothers to ensure that this foundation is as strong as possible so that our children may go on to live long and vibrant lives in good health.
(Catherine, integrative nutrition health coach)

Infection and Fever

Fever can appear rapidly with mild or severe symptoms, or slowly over the duration of an illness. Whatever way it presents itself, developing a fever means that your child's system is fighting to stay strong (producing more white blood cells), and to eradicate the offending bug (higher temperatures kill more germs). Rest and recuperation during this time is therefore recommended.

Remember, some sicknesses are simply part of growth and development, but having sound health during these times is helpful for quick recuperation and recovery.

Depending on the type of virus or infection they have, from the onset of symptoms your child is likely to be infectious and should stay home from school and away from friends, at least until they feel much better and the fever has disappeared. It is both unwise and unfair to allow your child to go about their normal activities during times of fever, as it poses not only a health risk to them, but to others also.

Time to Heal

Allow your child the time it takes to really recover and feel well again. If your child is still at an age where they cannot fully express their level of pain or discomfort, then ensuring plenty of recuperation is even more crucial. Just think back to a time when you yourself have been sick, and after thinking that you are better you go back to work or to the normal activity of life, then realise all too quickly that it was too soon. Imagine a child doing the same, who has missed school and their friends – he or she might not tell you if they begin to feel ill again. Imagine them trying to participate as normally as they can, studying, running in the playground; they might not know when to stop or slow down, until that it is, it is too late. It is at this point that the illness may return, more serious than before, and worse, that the immune system has now been compromised.

I understand how difficult it can be when one or more of your children are ill and you or your partner or loved ones need to take time away from your own job or social arrangements to tend to him or her, but offering genuine support during times of ill health is essential. Small children nearly always want their parents when they're sick, try to be there for them. Put work and other activities on hold as much as you can and spend a few days (more if needed) doing what it takes to keep your child comfortable. Allow your child to sleep and eat when they feel like it, distract them from their ailments and keep their spirits lifted. So much recent data points to the importance of remaining positive during times of illness (especially long-term chronic illness), and the part laughter and happiness has in boosting the immune system.

Strategies for Change:
- Strengthen your child's immune system by offering adequate rest and recuperation as needed.
- Consider alternatives to over-the-counter medicines that appeal to you.
- Distract your child from feelings of ill health by reading humorous stories or watching funny movies or cartoons together.

Food as Medicine

The basic principle of using food as medicine is that nutrients from foods can work in harmony with your body to keep it free from onset of injury or illness. As mentioned, your child will indeed suffer many normal and essential childhood illness; what I am speaking of here are the unnecessary, annoying maladies which upset the child and their lives on a more regular basis – colds, coughs, stomach upsets, hives and eczema for example.

From my own experiences with Jul, I quickly became aware of the fact that general health could be significantly boosted by the influence of good nutrition.

As a mother it is essential to proactively monitor your child's health. Why wait till your child is sick and suffering to treat them, and then only with medications that can mask symptoms and with repeated use, weaken the body? By making small but significant changes to your family's diet you are laying the foundation for prevention of illness. Put another way, you can be the influence on your child's future health.

Since the time I began weaning my first daughter I have always made sure that she has a healthy balanced diet, that includes lots of fresh fruits and vegetables, and I only ever let her drink water. Myself, and my husband are both healthy eaters so thankfully this has been easy for us to pass onto her. Fortunately she has never really suffered from colds or coughs, and is generally a healthy, happy child.
(Kelly, mother to daughters aged five and one)

As dramatic as it may sound, what your child eats will either prevent or provoke illness. Even as a number of outside influences barrage the body constantly and it is apparent that some of us have weaker immune systems than others, and indeed during times of illness we notice a decline. There is no doubt that a number of lifestyle choices, a poor diet being a major one, can be to blame.

The reason that some foods make our bodies sick and weaken the immune system is that they were not meant for human consumption in the first place, and if they are, then not always in the way that we are now producing them. A lot of food-like substances, chemicals and the like bombard many of our supermarket-shelf staples and in turn hinder proper absorption of real foods entering the body, and upset other important bodily processes and functions too. What I want you to think about is this: if food can cause us so much illness, then can't it also be the cure? If we educate ourselves properly, select nutrient-dense foods and remove the offending culprits that are making us sick, then won't it be true that real health is within our reach again? The answer is yes, and the wonderful thing about eating foods that are so nourishing is that the turn around from surviving to thriving is extremely quick!

> *Having a child with Down's syndrome made me even more aware of the importance of good nutrition. My son would catch every bug going around, so I did everything I could to keep his immune system strong through healthy diet and fresh produce, and no artificial flavours. The whole family is happier and healthier for eating wholefoods. As the children grew up they did not ask for or crave sweet and processed treats quite simply because they had them so rarely. Both my boys understand how good food makes you feel and less healthy choices can make you sick. I am confident that they will take their eating habits into adulthood.*
> *(Kerri, mother to sons aged sixteen and thirteen)*

By feeding your child a consistent, well-balanced diet (based primarily on nutrient content, as outlined in Chapter 2), you are fostering good dietary behaviours and tastes, and also strengthening the body as a whole. This simple act of maintaining healthy habits for your children will serve them well. If this alone isn't an immediate cure, ensuring a consistent and nourishing way of eating will at the very least put the body in a better position to take care of itself.

> *For myself and my family I see diet and lifestyle as one of the first areas to address if our health is not optimum. From general fatigue and feeling unwell, and I believe to more severe conditions and chronic disease, nutrition can help immeasurably.*
> *(Jacqueline, mother to daughters aged three and one)*

If your child is fortunate to be generally healthy (and is rarely sick), it is still important to pay close attention to what they eat because consuming a wholesome diet is essential to preventing future ill health. If I had not had Jul first I would have pretty much breezed through the first few years of my other two sons' lives and never experienced the pain, worry and frustration that we did. They, in contrast to Jul, nursed for two years, only started on solids after seven months, and ate pretty much anything and everything that I offered them. They didn't suffer from allergies, slept well and were generally easy-going. The point is that even though a child is healthy (and we hope continues to be), that doesn't mean that you should take that for granted. We don't always know the reasons why one child is born sick and another isn't, why one is a picky eater while others devour everything, why some breeze through childhood illness and others suffer. What we do know is that maintaining a healthy diet will assist their development in a wide range of areas and being able to provide your child with the opportunity to carry their health into adulthood is a gift that I would like to see every child receive.

Eating with the Seasons

The importance of eating seasonally unfortunately seems to be a well-kept secret that a lot of families are missing out on. In one of my favourite go-to books, John Douillard, Ayurvedic doctor and father to six children, writes, *eat the foods that are provided by the harvest of the season. There is a relationship between foods and the time of year they ripen naturally. Each harvest offers medicinal benefits to protect us from that season's maladies.* (J.Douillard, *Perfect Health for Kids,* 2004.)

> *We have proven to ourselves as a family the importance of healthy eating. We moved to a new home, stopped some of our regular habits; we ate out more, and succumbed to new tempting treats. We lived in temporary housing, and then once we moved into our own house we were without a kitchen for month, so we were all out of our routine. Both of our kids are now sick with flu and were sick for the whole of last month too. We know what we should be doing; it's just challenging once you let things slip. We will all get there again, because we all know how much more energetic, happy and healthy we feel when we are feeding ourselves properly.*
> *(Michael, father to children aged fifteen and twelve)*

Know Your Environment

Not only will the seasons directly impact the local foods available to you and how they can positively improve health, interpreting your own location's weather and climate patterns are significant too.

Living in a dry, dusty and hot atmosphere can offset a completely different set of health concerns compared to residing somewhere damp and cold. Knowing your environment and how the seasons will affect your family's health will give you the time to prepare in order to prevent unnecessary illness. For example, in hotter parts of the world where I have lived the weather during many months can be extremely warm and very drying. It is during these months that I ensure that my children drink extra water, eat foods with a higher water content, wear sunscreen whenever they are outdoors, bathe in oil to prevent dry skin, use natural oils in their nose to prevent sinus problems, take off extra clothing when outdoors but remember to replace when inside air-conditioned buildings. This may sound like a long list but it's just a few extra steps in your day that quickly become habitual, and particularly when your child is at a young and vulnerable age, each and every measure you take can really make a difference in keeping your child comfortable and well.

> *Every little helps. I watch my wife and acknowledge that each and every practice is going in some small way towards supporting and sustaining the far bigger picture of our children's health.*
> *(My husband)*

Medicinal Foods

Garlic
We all should have garlic in the kitchen, and find ways to use it when preparing our family's meals. Allicin is the compound in garlic that is recognised for its health benefits on the body. Consuming garlic is understood to boost the immune system in a number of powerful ways.

Ginger
Ginger is most commonly known for its spicy taste and its anti-inflammatory benefits. Ginger can be used to ease an upset stomach and the symptoms associated with sickness, especially nausea. Juicing ginger in with your regular juice, or cooking this root in a warm drink or soup can also help to combat a sore throat.

Local Honey
Raw, local honey has many benefits. Its ability to ward off and even prevent allergies is widely praised and is known as immunotherapy. The idea is that you get a small amount of the thing you might be allergic to, which can, over time, reduce your symptoms.

I first learned about the amazing properties and benefits of manuka honey and turmeric at a lecture on Ayurveda during my nutrition training. Ayurvedic medicine, founded in India, is one of the world's oldest holistic practices.

Manuka honey
Another natural anti-inflammatory, produced by bees pollinating the native manuka

bush. Manuka honey can be used to make a medicinal paste (see Tried and Tested At Home Formulas), eaten with other foods, and can also be used topically for minor wounds and burns.

Turmeric (the bright orange spice we use mostly in curries).
With its main active ingredient curcumin, has long been hailed as nature's antibiotic, a powerful anti-inflammatory and antioxidant and is believed to have anti-cancer properties.

Hydration

Staying hydrated is generally considered a vital component of overall health. While it might seem obvious, depending on your child's daily diet, activity levels, climate and any recent illness, maintaining adequate levels can at times be difficult. A good indicator of hydration is checking to see if your child's pee is the right colour. A normal range will be indicated by a clear to very pale yellow colour with no offensive smell, while deeper colour and more intense smell suggest that additional amounts of fluids are needed. It is not unusual for the first pee of the day to be slightly darker in colour, due to the long hours that a child may have slept, but darker urine during the day could warrant concern. The very best liquid for your child is still, clean water, drunk at regular intervals throughout the day. Unlike other beverages, water will not spoil a child's appetite, so happily offer it at the dinner table too. Offer small amounts of water to babies as soon as they start on solids, and for the whole family only ever place water in your portable water carriers. Sucking on juice (even fresh) too often can cause serious tooth decay.

Constipation

Although it may be difficult to identify the exact cause of your child's constipation, dehydration can be a significant factor. Other ways to help prevent, or at the very least to alleviate some of the uncomfortable symptoms your child may experience, include consuming enough fibre (found in fresh fruits and vegetables) and eating whole grains (found in cereals and rice), helping your child feel as comfortable as possible when using the toilet, and staying active with regular exercise. It is also worth pointing out that a recent upset or sudden change to your child's eating habits or routine can also contribute to the factors that cause constipation.

To Supplement or Not

While vitamins and minerals in the form of supplements might be necessary for the short term to recuperate from ill health, they should *always* be prescribed by a medical professional. If you or your family member feels lacking in some vital nutrient I urge you to look further than a bottle of pills, firstly by ensuring through a series of simple blood tests that there is not a more serious medical issue that needs addressing. From there, you can look to your daily diet to ensure that no vital element is missing. If you are unsure of how to do this, try keeping a food diary – it really is an excellent way to keep track of what you are *really* eating (or, as is often the case, what you are *not* eating).

Something to Think About

It is generally considered safer to get all the vitamins and minerals you need naturally from the foods you consume. Dietary sources not only contain higher, more natural amounts of the vitamin or mineral you might be missing, but are far better absorbed by the body in this way. Supplement distributors may give us the impression that a single vitamin can cure or ward off an illness, but administered alone, without careful consideration of one's whole diet, it is simply not possible.

Probiotics

Probiotics, also known as good bacteria are found naturally in the body and help to keep the gut healthy. Some people are born simply not having enough; others will suffer depletion due to poor diet or overuse of antibiotics, causing an individual to feel unwell. Regular probiotic supplementation is considered safe for your child and particularly advisable during, or after antibiotic treatment, however, you might opt to incorporate fermented foods known for their probiotic properties as well as or instead. An easy one to find and include (if your child is not lactose sensitive) is natural yoghurt (with active or live cultures). Other powerful fermented choices that you might like to research and try with your child include kefir, kimchi, kombucha tea, miso, sauerkraut and tempeh. These options may be new or sound foreign to you, but select one or two that appeal to you and your family, and add them in where you can.

Strategies for Change:

- Consider foods as medicine the next time your child is poorly.
- Keep individual water bottles accessible for each member of your family (you will be surprised at how often they reach for them when they are nearby).
- Start offering a wider variety of foods to ensure your family are getting a host of vital vitamins and minerals.

Prevention = Cure

There was once a time when I took my children to the doctor as soon as they complained of an ailment or accident. Despite my trust in the system available to me I have learned to evaluate the situation first. Being your family's health advocate will not only save you time and money, but will allow you to play an active role in the decision-making process. As a mother you should go armed with the questions and concerns that you have for your child, and work alongside the doctor to reach an agreeable prescription to aid recovery of the illness.

Regardless of the qualifications that a doctor holds, and not to mention the wealth of experience he or she has, you should remember that their say does not have to be final. It is easy to feel anxious when your child is sick, desperate for a diagnosis and a way to heal them. Even though it may be the obvious signs and symptoms that your doctor is looking at, it is usually the underlying indicators that only you will know as a parent that really help to get to the bottom of what is *really* going on, so try to remain confident.

If you feel you can speak frankly with your child's doctor you are off to a great start. It is essential at this meeting to feel comfortable asking questions and seeking clarification on anything that you don't understand. There is nothing worse than sitting mute, coming home, and wishing you had asked this or that question, or even why a particular diagnosis or medicine was given.

Something to Think About

Keeping a diary of why and when your child is sick will help you communicate better with your doctor and other health professionals whom you may see or seek out in the future.

After many long and complicated conversations with our children's paediatrician, brought on by Jul's complications over the years, I feel we have created a very relaxed connection where we can communicate openly. We both know that our shared concern is one of mutual care for and loyalty to my children, his patients. Unlike many doctors I have met, our current paediatrician does not cut me off when I explain to him my child's symptoms, he does not presume he knows more than I do about my child, he is positively welcoming of my suggestions and my questions, and helps me to fully understand what he is thinking, diagnosing and ultimately prescribing. If you have not been made to feel this way, as tricky as it might be, it is time to find your family another medical professional.

> *It is very important for me as a doctor to establish a comfortable and trusting relationship with my patients' parents or caregivers. I learn so much more about the child with their cooperation.*
> *(Dr Ammer, paediatrician and father to four children)*

If your child has to spend a period of time in hospital then communicating with those who are taking care of your child will be even more important. Time spent in hospital can be extremely stressful for all concerned, and your sick child will need your support and comfort now more than ever. Please read my sister's advice in the Professional's Comments at the end of this chapter for ways to cope.

The Issue With Weight

As I look back on the birth weights and body structure of my first two boys, they couldn't be more different. Jul was born long and thin, and is now lean and very strong, athletic and prone to losing weight easily. Sahm, on the other hand, was a heavy baby, always fed very heartily, and is more heavyset and rounded now, and less active than his brother. Of course I cannot put it down to what they eat alone, because just like your children each one will need different dietary requirements based on their likes and dislikes, energy levels, age and a host of other factors. What some doctors fail to look at is the background of your child. From the time your baby is born doctors will tell you how they rate according to a growth chart. This chart does not take into account if your child is breastfed or not, and certainly doesn't look at ethnicity or family traits that have been inherited. Jul has taken on many of the qualities from my side of the family and Sahm from his father's. What I feel is more important for the doctor to look at is whether the child is growing steadily, if they are continuing to put on weight and height, if they are strong, eating well, sleeping well and physically active, if they have good fine and gross motor skills for their age – the list goes on…

I couldn't be more put off by a health professional who is only concerned about my child gaining weight, because as we all know there is an extremely fine line between being a good and healthy weight and becoming over weight. I was once told by a doctor that I should feed Jul up to ten tablespoons of olive oil a day, and that I should let him feast on greasy foods such as hamburgers and fries. I couldn't believe what I was hearing! This advice was, of course, terrible, and knowing better I didn't follow it, but what about for those parents who don't know, and do follow such instructions? I would rather have my child maintain a stable weight from eating a host of fresh and wholesome foods that I know are helping him to thrive, rather than from a range of undesirable foods groups that will inevitably help him to gain weight, but will in the long term have direct negative implications on the rest of his growing mind and body.

Childhood Obesity

According to the public health advocate, Marion Nestle, PhD, child nutrition was once focused on dietary insufficiency, whereas today the most serious problem is childhood obesity, and the health and social issues directly related to it. (M. Nestle, *Food Politics*, 2007.)

Just as some of you might be finding it hard to help your son or daughter put on weight, others are finding it just as difficult to help theirs lose unwanted pounds. As your child ages they will go through periods of transition and adjustment. Your youngster will begin to spend more time and energy at school and in sports, and very likely more time away from home and from you. They will begin to make many of their own food choices, and without education, prior supervision and above all peer pressure (not forgetting genuine hunger from all the activities they are pursuing), eating some unhealthy foods is now quite common and can lead to losing or adding extra weight. The manner in which you approach your child and their changing body will make all the difference to him or her, accepting him- or herself.

This is the point where everything else you read in NOURISH and put into place will help you to help your child. Education is key, support is essential and nourishment is vital. Despite popular media coverage in support of plus size and being comfortable 'as you are', it is imperative to understand that it is unhealthy to be overweight (and of course underweight), and both have adverse effects on the body as a whole. What's more important is being healthy for your individual body type, and this is something that I wish social media pursued much more.

> *As a family we structure conversations around making healthy choices by using terms such as 'being kind to our body' rather than negative language about body image and physical appearance. With two daughters aged nine and thirteen years, we are very careful to communicate in a way that does not refer to being 'fat' or 'thin', but rather steer them towards a lifestyle that allows for them to make their own conscious choices.*
> *(Katie, mother to children aged fifteen, thirteen and nine)*

Despite your best intentions to aid your child who is longing for a body that is not their own, support them through the healthy habits that have been written about here. If you have raised your child in a loving and supportive home, help them to find their way back to healthy habits and lifestyle pursuits. No matter what you do, unless it is a medical emergency never dramatically decrease or increase their food intake. Children at any age are growing more than we can imagine, and a child being deprived or stuffed with food will only lead them to make unhealthy comparisons with diets and their image. Instead, increase the amount of nutrients in their food. When a child is nutrient full the body learns genuine hunger and satisfaction all by itself.

> *To have life in your body, you must have life in your food.*
> *(Hippocrates Health Institute)*

Malnutrition

It may seem absurd to speak about your child being malnourished, but it can certainly happen. For some people living in places in the world where quality food is difficult to come by, or for those who are living on an extremely tight food budget, malnutrition is certainly a threat, but what about for those of you who do spend considerable amounts of money on shopping and/or have access to a whole range of foods for your family?

Malnutrition is not always about starvation. The truth is that many overweight people are malnourished and suffering. A definition that I use describes it as a lack of proper nutrition. This can unquestionably be caused by under-eating, but not eating enough of the right stuff causes many more of the cases seen today. If we continually feed our children food that lacks adequate nutrition, the body is compromised, and in due course the immune system is put under serious strain and is broken down, resulting in illness and eventual disease.

Everything in Moderation?

When I work with clients to help them achieve optimum health I am regularly asked, 'Well, isn't it OK to eat everything in moderation?' Can some unhealthy foods be considered part of a balanced diet? That, of course, depends on the individual diet of your family, and what you personally consider and accept moderation to be. Eating processed foods once a week might be considered acceptable in one household; eating them every day considered OK, in another. Your decisions, I believe (and I have seen), will be very much based on education and what you learn about the foods you are eating and how they affect your family's health.

Your child's body will almost certainly cry out for what it needs the most, but interpreting this can be difficult. This is where your role of encouraging variety is central to creating a healthy eater.

Cravings

Foreseeing a dip in blood sugar (hunger) creeping up on your child can also be difficult to manage, which is why the task of feeding them with nutrition in mind is key. If hunger does strike due to missed meals or foods lacking nutrition, your child may favour foods that are less than desirable, purely because at this point they are looking for instant gratification (and as adults, we know all too well how that feels!). Suddenly craving something sweet leads you to irrationally choose the chocolate bar instead of the apple, simple protein snack or smoothie, for example. It may be difficult to wrestle with your child's emotions at this point but do try to stand steadfast on giving them something that will truly satisfy their hunger.

As I have just touched upon, cravings can be detrimental to one's health; they can monopolise the diet and regularly threaten a person's best efforts to eat better. Cravings, however, despite the negative impact they can have, also alert us to imbalance within the body and can pinpoint us towards those foods we might be missing, and that are good for us.

It is necessary to highlight here the major causes of cravings. Dehydration can be one, which is why it's so important not to mistake thirst for hunger. Nutrient deficiency is another, due to a lack of vital vitamins and minerals being absorbed through your current diet, and hormonal imbalance and emotions, where we overindulge in comfort foods normally associated with a positive experience. Another common cause of craving that we vastly overlook is the consequence of craving more of the foods you are eating most often. We can see this clearly in the child who eats an abundance of sweets, then asks for more sugar.

Physical Activity

Being physically active is a huge deterrent for ill health, and something that comes very naturally to the young child is their physical ability and agility. As soon as a toddler can, they are up and running, climbing, jumping, hardly stopping for a moment, maybe only to eat, rest and sleep. This type of activity aids the growth of your developing child, forming strong bones, enhancing lung power and supporting the immune system. Vigorous activity increases the appetite and promotes healthy eating.

I notice with Jul that after a long day at school and his after-school activities he is just happy to have food to come home to. Gone are his picky tendencies; he seldom seeks for what he *wants* any more, just what he *needs*. With all the demands on his growing body, physically, mentally and socially, his needs are changing. It appears that his hunger knows how it wants to be fed, with nourishing, nutrient-dense, life-supporting foods.

As your child starts to grow up and become more interested in formal sports, steer them towards activities that they have a natural ability for, and of course hobbies that they like and can have fun with. Being physically active encourages good health practices and makes your child aware of what the human body needs and what it is capable of.

> *Being physically active and participating in sports is built into our family culture.*
> *We all play and support each other by going to each other's games and events.*
> *I ensure that full participation from everyone is a priority.*
> *(Preet, mother to children aged ten and eight)*

Strategies for Lasting Change:

- If you feel as if a family member has a strong yearning for one food or another, keep a food journal for a number of days (three to seven) to see the patterns within the diet and to acknowledge which foods or ingredients are causing the cravings.

- If you suspect a particular food or ingredient is to blame, you must replace it before you remove it completely. For example, if sugar is the culprit, replace processed foods with the wholefood alternatives: processed jams and jellies for 100%fruit varieties, cookies for your home-made and more wholesome ones, fresh fruit instead of canned – the list goes on.

- Offer and encourage a cornucopia of foods from every food group. Eating in this way will ensure that your child, and indeed your whole family, will get the very best of what they need, leaving very little room for deficiencies.

Professional's Comments: Nikki Kenmore, Registered Nurse, Child Branch

As a nurse in a hospital setting, how important do you think the relationship is between child, nurse and doctor and parent, nurse and doctor?

It is vital. The three-way relationship is essential for the patient's care and recovery. It is beneficial for the both the nurse and doctor to gain the confidence and respect of both the child and parent and the other way around, as all parties hold vital information to help aid the child's diagnosis, medical care and recuperation.

Patients and parents can feel intimated in a hospital setting. As a health professional what would your advice be to parents with sick children?

With little to no exception the parent or child's main caregiver will always know more about the child's history and must be encouraged to vocalise and actively participate with the child's medical staff or team. Everyone who is tending to your child will do their utmost to care for him or her appropriately, but I do know that in some circumstances families find it difficult to comprehend prognosis and diagnosis due to emotional stress and lack of understanding. If information is too general please don't be afraid to ask for further explanation or speak with a nurse who you can depend upon. Nurses will often act as a 'bridge' between patient or parent and doctor(s) if one feels unconfident, is nervous to speak up, or is led or made to feel uncomfortable.

As a parent, what would your advice be?

As fraught and as difficult as watching your sick child in hospital can be, try as much as you can to stay focused and dependable, at the very least when you are in front of your child. The hospital setting can be an overwhelming and scary place for them, and seeing you assert yourself and staying calm when they are not will reassure them and make medical procedures easier.

If a parent felt it was needed, where would one seek out additional support for their child?

Depending on the complexities of your child's current health he or she may already have or been referred to a multi-disciplinary team. Doctors who feel it necessary to seek additional support will appropriately signpost to other doctors and/or therapists who can join your child's medical team to offer specialised advice and treatment. If you are in any doubt as to whether your child requires additional care you are perfectly within your right to ask. Instead of asking, for example, 'Does my child need to see a dietician?' try, 'Why doesn't my child need to see a dietician?' This way you are given more than a one-word answer, and the doctor should satisfy your questioning by providing you with a measurable answer that is convincing.

For a child's recovery, how important do you think it is for them to receive care and attention in addition to medical assistance?
It is critical. When a child is shown care, understanding, encouragement and support they will get better quicker. A child should be made as comfortable as possible and acknowledged for who they are, not just for the sickness that they have.

As a mother to one young son, what advice can you offer on ways to maintain health?
Try as much as you can to promote a clean and safe environment for your child. Set realistic boundaries through loving encouragement, by offering appealing foods, and by supporting healthy habits and behaviours by displaying them yourself. Notice your child, know their habits and likes and dislikes, and pay attention to any changes. Look out for signs and symptoms that your child is unwell, and when appropriate keep them away from regular activities if they are suffering from or recovering from sickness, and provide them with on-going education so they too can learn how to prevent illness and maintain good health.

Something else I would like to add is not to rely too heavily on the Internet. Especially if you are researching signs and symptoms, the Internet can prove misleading. Although it is a wonderful tool to provide you with insightful information and guidance once you have a diagnosis, seek out a trusted health care provider in the meantime.

Health – Your Questions Answered

There have been times when my child doesn't eat as well or as much as I would like. Should I be worried?

Try to remember that your child will not actually starve him- or herself. Unless your child has a medical condition that needs to be taken care of, children go through periods in their young lives where they go off their food. Teething, times of sickness, emotions or a change in routine can all affect a child's eating habits and patterns. Try to stay as relaxed as you can during these times, do not force food upon your child, support these transitions and they will eventually eat and drink what they need to – the body has a remarkable way of letting them know. I absolutely understand that these times can be stressful but please know that like many other growing pains, this time will pass. If you are at all worried then do visit a trusted paediatrician or general practitioner to put your mind at rest.

My child's school frowns upon time taken for being absent due to illness; tell me this isn't the norm?

This is definitely a sore subject of mine. Whilst I clearly understand the need for children to be at school as much as they can, days taken off due to illness, feelings of malaise or physical injury are indeed warranted. What I feel the school should be more concerned about is the number of children who are attending school while they are sick, and those who are coming back to school too soon. Such cases are putting other children at risk and are prolonging the life of simple viruses that are quick to spread but easy to contain if treated correctly.

My son recently suffered weight loss due to sickness. What can I do to help him regain the lost kilos?

My best advice would be to feed him as normally as he will let you and be patient. During this recovery time remember that his immune system may still be weak, and probably his body is still a little tired from being ill. You can certainly offer him healthy, known weight-gaining foods like avocado, nuts, whole-grains and more, but in general just feeding him a diet based on a broad selection of nutritious foods will help him get back on track.

Chapter 5

FOCUS ON NURTURE

Just as you are transforming your own life, may you transform
the lives of those around you.
(Paolo Coelho)

To nurture sums up all the ways in which I hope to be a good mother. Even with all the complexities of pregnancy, childbirth, breastfeeding, sleeplessness, illness and the general worry that comes with being a new parent, mothers remain dedicated to nurturing their young. Mothers of all ages and ethnicities have one thing in common: that innate feeling to safeguard and care for their child. You become like a mother bear; intensely committed to protecting her cub, no matter what.

To nurture your child means you will try incredibly hard to encourage, cherish and support all aspects of your child's developing life. As you resolve to raise a healthy child, think about what sort of commitment you will make to him or her and the rest of your family. What type of lifestyle will you offer, model and foster? You have the power to take the necessary steps towards preventing poor health and preserving a life of well-being.

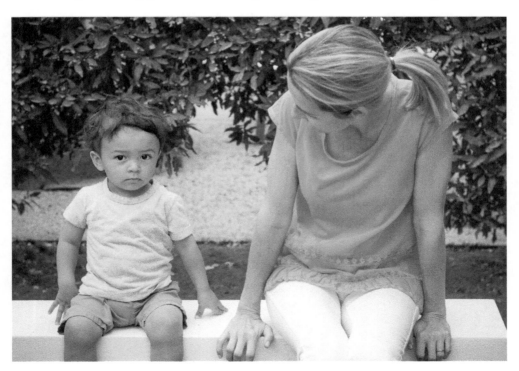

Motherhood

One of the greatest challenges facing any mother is raising her family and doing it well. The debate over whether to stay at home, work from home, or work outside the home is complex and depends on a huge number of factors. Whatever your situation, your role as a mother will include many duties.

While fathers undoubtedly play a huge role in the family circle, statistically they spend more time working away from the home, often resulting in mothers being responsible for the care of the house, food selection and cooking, and the mammoth task of children's everyday needs and wants. You may ask at this point how realistic it is, then, to model and promote health in the many areas that are required? It will indeed be a challenge to begin with, but a necessary priority. As a mother, you have been given the gift of raising your child. As you think about implementing these principles, feel empowered knowing that your efforts will also be your greatest rewards.

> *There are not many things you can control in life – life is going to happen, the good and the bad, no matter what you do. One thing you can hope to steer, to a large extent, is the development of your child through the health choices you make for them. As a mother, you can only protect your children in limited ways for a limited time, but a healthy body will surely protect them for the rest of their lives and long after they leave your loving arms.*
> *(Catherine, mother to daughter aged four)*

Whether your family's journey to health has been established (yet needs support or improving), not quite yet (but you mean to start) or somewhere in between, make a vow right now to commit with determination to bring forth change.

In the Beginning

As you can probably guess, an ideal place to start would be at the beginning, from the birth and the subsequent months and years with your child. Starting from here allows you to condition your child's health and eating habits much more closely, but please have confidence that this is not everyone's journey (as a first-time mother it was certainly not mine). Begin from where you can; it is never too late.

Easy Does It

It is all too easy to get caught up and overexcited with a new routine in your family's life. While the immediate action may be necessary and is indeed to be commended, do remember to implement change slowly, particularly when it affects the whole family. Apply yourself carefully, ensuring that all members of the family are fully informed of each adjustment. For example, if you are trying out new recipes, let others help, and if you are replacing less desirable foods with more nutritious ones, know that this transition may take some time. Be patient and continue to model, encourage and explain to your family the reasons why adopting change will benefit them.

> *Healthy eating and living keeps the whole family well and happy.*
> *When I was younger I educated myself on good eating habits and now as a mother,*
> *I feel empowered that I get to pass along these lessons and values to my son.*
> *(Meeka, mother to son aged nine)*

Shared Decision Making

Recruit the help of your children; it will make the entire process of change much simpler. Children have shared rights in my home, where I encourage them to voice their opinions and get involved. By providing your child with the opportunities to share thoughts and make some of the decisions, you are showing them how valued they are and how effective their ideas can be.

Something to Think About

I believe that children value one-on-one time as one of the most important things you can offer them. Dedicated time with your child will show them just how special they are, and just how serious *you* are about them being able to receive the information you are giving.

Your Significant Other

Being able to count on the support of your significant other, whether this is your husband, a close family member or friend, will prove instrumental as you go forward. Having someone to back you up when you implement change will demonstrate to the rest of your family the sincerity of what you are trying to achieve. I know for me having my husband by my side as I introduce new health concepts to our boys has been confirmation of his faith in all that I am doing. Having him reiterate why said health practice or choice of foods is important to our sons is so reassuring and allows me to take a step back when I cannot be around.

Family Support

You and your extended family members may not have exactly the same views when it comes to what you feed your children. However, it is imperative that you convey just how important it is for them to understand, respect and continue with certain food choices when the children are in their care. If at first they don't agree or understand, take the time to sit down and talk about how your new food choices are really benefiting your children, or offer them some simple but informative material that will explain your reasons more clearly. My mother actually prefers that I tell her (or bring with me) exactly what my boys can eat – that way the decisions are taken care of and she can spend more time enjoying them. My father secretly tells me that he is going to feed my children junk food, but I know he wouldn't dare! He is actually very healthy himself, active and eats well, and is more of a role model to my boys than he knows.

If you have a child minder, nanny or other employed persons that work in your home, with your child, communicate with them constantly. It is crucial with carers that they fully understand the requirements you have for your child.

Model for Success

If you didn't know it already, take note that you are very likely your child's biggest influence. You may not have thought to what extent your child is watching and copying you, but if you think about it, it is quite impossible for them not to. You are their provider and, therefore, their guide. From the onset of implementing healthy change it might seem difficult, especially if your child has already picked up some unhealthy habits, but as you begin to become more health-aware and increase your own understanding, have the confidence to know that you are on the right path. The success you will surely notice from implementing new habits will motivate you to keep going.

I believe the best way for a mother to drive children towards a healthy lifestyle is to be their role model. Going through some unexpected experiences in my life means that I have learned that keeping myself healthy and setting the right examples for my kids is extremely important.
(Fatima, mother to children aged nine and seven)

For me personally, seeing my children well, and wanting them to continue in this way, is reason and incentive enough to practise and promote a healthy lifestyle. Despite there being a number of excellent role models available for my children, I also worry about the influence of the ones who are not so ideal (as discussed in Chapter 1). If kids have someone in their very own home to watch and to learn from, someone who is looking out for their best interests and future, a parent in my opinion is by far one of the greatest choices there is.

You Learn as They Grow

With Jul, in the early years, I don't think I really trusted myself enough as a mother. I was afraid to do anything on my own, I was always seeking others' advice and approval, and I did everything too quickly, especially around offering food, particularly among others. I just wanted to fit in. Fast-forward through the years, and with my subsequent children, I am much firmer with myself because I have learned from my mistakes, and because I now know how vital the health of my children is. I have my own set of standards now, and I am very much set on sticking to them.

I feel that as a mother who practises health for herself, I am modelling daily the choices my children can make in their own lives to be healthy. I am allowing them the chance to grow with good nutrition and exercise so that their minds and bodies are programmed to function in a healthy way from a young age. As a family, finding joy and connection through healthy choices and activities brings us closer together and allows all of us to be a support and positive reinforcement for healthy choices.
(Yvonne, mother to children aged eight and six)

Practise What You Preach

As a parent responsible for raising your child, it is imperative to show them the way, and not just tell them. Children can be confused if a lesson or message you are trying to convey is not consistent or clear, or is lacking integrity. This can lead to a lack of respect, or worse, to them rejecting your ideas and/or efforts entirely. Let us look at some examples that display this type of contradiction: a mother lecturing her child on eating healthy foods, yet regularly eats junk food; a child being scolded for copying the actions of an adult who is smoking and told this is only something you do when you are older; or when you force your child to partake in an activity they don't enjoy, but make no effort to show them how fun it is.

By demonstrating genuine practices of health yourself, you can help your child to do the same. Even if at first this is only exhibited at home, as long as the message is consistent it is an excellent place to start.

> *Be consistent, like any good routine it needs to happen most of the time not some of the time.*
> *(Charlotte, mother to sons aged six and three)*

The Family Dinner Table

The dinner table is a place full of possibilities to both nurture and nourish your family. As a parent typically responsible for the feeding of your family, that means creating an environment that is favourable to your health beliefs. Start by aiming to establish your own family customs around eating.

For me, I have brought many rituals from my own childhood, yet my husband and I have also started some of our own. No matter how small the meal, make a habit of sitting at the dining or kitchen table. Sitting around a table, undisturbed by the TV, phone or other annoyances, will allow your family to enjoy the food and this time together.

I witness with my own children how much they enjoy the intimacy of this family setting, and how much more willing they are to accept or try new foods as we talk about and sample them together. Sitting down and eating together has long been proven to be a wonderful way to promote healthy family relationships, and for some families it may be the only time of the day when you all come together. I know that as my children grow up this family tradition we have created will considerably benefit them and their love for one another and for good food.

Something to Think About
You can recreate dinner table rituals in other settings. From time to time my family will

eat in our back garden, take a picnic to the park or even create a picnic indoors. As long as you continue with nutritious choices, not each and every mealtime has to be the same.

Removing Negative Connections

The importance of creating a safe haven around meals is paramount for all children but especially those who have built up negative connections to food. Children who express stress during mealtimes through sadness, anger or frustration will create an emotional connection with the food they are being offered and are likely to reject it. On the other hand, children who experience joy, fun and inclusion at the dinner table will make a positive connection to that same food and happily consume it. Children need to sense a parent's approval and genuine understanding, and feel comfortable with the way mealtimes are handled. Give your child the autonomy he or she deserves at this young, sensitive age, and have tolerance for and faith in your child.

Having Patience With Change

Having the patience you need to reinforce healthy habits with your child at the dining table can be difficult. Let's be frank, it can be stressful, especially if you have more than one child and their different likes and dislikes to contend with. However, it is very much up to the parents in the family to set the tone at mealtimes, and to sincerely welcome your child to the table, making it a safe place where your children always feel included. Never force-feed, exclude, argue with or punish your child at the dinner table, but do set clear boundaries and attainable expectations. Offer on-going encouragement and in due time, your child will enjoy coming to the table and eating there.

Primary Food

At Integrative Nutrition®, the largest nutrition school in the world, through which I spent the most amazing year distance learning, I was introduced to the concept of Primary Food™. *The philosophy about food is that everything we consider as a source of nutrition is really just a secondary source of nourishment.* The foods we consume are actually secondary to other important aspects of our life, those that provide us with energy, in particular relationships and physical activity (and as we age also spirituality and career). A positive relationship with your child, therefore, one that they can really rely upon and enjoy, is vital to helping them develop a safe connection with what they eat. If your child is not fulfilled by their primary foods they may look to food, as so many do, as complete nourishment and not as something that simply fuels them. *The more primary food we give ourselves, the less we depend on secondary food. On the contrary, the more we fill ourselves with secondary food, the less space we leave for primary food.* (www.integrativenutrition. com)

> *Give your child as much love and support as they need. Being a strong, united family is also important.*
> *(Emma, mother to children aged three and one)*

Positive Reinforcement

At an immature age children will seek the attention of those special adults in their lives because it feels good. This can often be seen at mealtimes, where they are regularly being asked to sit down and conform. Children are generally looking for positive attention, but sometimes try to draw a negative reaction that can also be rewarding for them. As hard as it can be, try not to give in to the negative emotions, distract your child from this behaviour, take a deep breath if you need to, and continue with the support and encouragement as always.

I was reminded last night of the huge role an older sibling can play in order to reinforce positive eating habits and behaviours at the dinner table. If your child has an older brother or sister, cousins, extended relatives or good friends who regularly join your family to eat, use this difference in age and maturity to your advantage. There will be times when I don't even have to remind or caution my middle child to eat another bite or try this or that food because his brother will have done it already. Indeed, more often than not he is happy to. After all, it must get a little boring for children to be prompted on how to do this and that by their parents all of the time, and so to have someone close in age, who they look up to, to assist and encourage them will be nice.

Tools for Success

There are a number of books and online resources to help you educate and support your child around eating better. I tend to reach out to these at times other than when we are actually eating, when I see that one of my boys is having a hard time with transitioning to a new food or struggling at the table. What I actually love to do is use my son's favourite book or movie character (right now, for Sahm it's the Hulk) and tell stories of what foods make him strong and able to defeat the bad guys. Once we are seated at the dinner table again I can give snippets of these stories to remind him of the habits we are trying to achieve. Not only do these tales offer him a distraction that allows me to help him eat his meals more easily, he is genuinely entertained and further educated because of them.

Do remember that even young children can help with mealtime preparations. Have them set the table alongside you, help them to choose or make their very own place mats and purchase cutlery that is playful or otherwise age-appropriate for them to use.

Eating With Hands

It is not uncommon for young babies to take their very first bite of their very first food using their bare hands. The texture and smell of a certain food are very important to a child experimenting with taste, so please allow them to do this. Eating will, at first, be very messy, so be prepared, but watch how your young child delights in trying new foods! Of course as a mother, we can hope to expect that in time, our child will feed him- or herself quite happily using utensils, and this you can certainly help with; just don't rush it along faster than you need to. All my boys, in spite of their differing ages, continue to eat almost all of their snacks with their hands and very much take pleasure in doing so.

Reap What You Sow

Being able to delight in your child's successes won't always come easily, and don't expect it to. You will see some children take to each and every food enthusiastically while others will need guidance, your complete backing and most of all, your time.

From the start with Jul, his on-going illness meant that almost anything and everything we fed him managed to upset him in some way. He was plagued with hives, would gag when offered food with a particular texture, and seemed to debate over whether he wanted to eat much of anything at all. Yet, through perseverance, a lot of understanding, education and family support, Jul started to become more interested in and to relish his food. For the past five years, Jul has been encouraged to eat almost anything we offer him and now voices his opinion over his choices for a meal, snack, and even restaurants. It is with pride that I watch this boy devour (and love) home-made juices, protein-packed smoothies, muffins, and bread – I could go on and on… oh, and a mammoth plate of mixed raw and fruits and vegetables every day!

Strategies for Change:

- If our children are set to imitate us, then give them someone and something positive to imitate. Knowing that you are your child's role model will hopefully spur you on to maintain healthy habits for yourself.
- Enjoy your food. Children who see their parent(s) eating nutritious foods with enthusiasm sense the joy, then do the same.
- When possible, have all members of your family sitting at the dinner table for meals. The inclusion of everyone shows your child(ren) the significance of this family tradition.

Social Acceptance

Did you know that being social not only increases the quality and even length of life, but adds to overall well-being too? What better reason, then, for you and your family to maintain great relationships with family and friends? Eating with others is one particular social arrangement that as families we have been partaking in for years. Preparing, cooking, baking, sharing, offering and consuming meals provides a chance to practise togetherness, as well as an excellent way of demonstrating healthy habits to be passed down from one generation to another.

Social Eating

As socially important as eating is, the food choices your children are faced with won't always be agreeable, particularly those outside of the home. Children's parties and celebrations have sadly become notorious for serving junk foods, and the influence of this is often unavoidable. With my own children, I tend to include them in the choice and preparation of foods that we will be having and sharing with our friends. When they do take an interest in junk or party foods, especially if others are eating them, despite my own reservations I understand fully their intrigue, and so if my child should ask I allow them to take a few bites and further encourage them to eat what we have brought, or something else that is nutritious. Now that my children have grown used to me preparing snacks, and most junk foods are still unavailable to them, they rarely ask for something different.

> *I worry that my kids are often affected by seeing their friends choose the unhealthy foods they are not permitted to eat.*
> *(Amy, mother to children aged seven and five)*

If I am really keen for my children to avoid a particular food – for example, fizzy drinks or something else equally processed – then I simply explain that this is something that we as a family have chosen to exclude from our diet. I remind them gently of the many ways in which we are trying to stay healthy, but offer them the chance to recreate something similar at home – freshly prepared lemonade, perhaps? I know all too well that the time will come when I will not be so able to negotiate or steer every choice my boys make, and I don't want to. By providing them with alternatives and raising them to appreciate a healthy lifestyle, I feel confident that they will make these choices themselves.

At a recent holiday party I was shocked by the generous amounts of soft drinks made available to the kids. I knew that if the drinks had not been available, the children would have asked for water, and been perfectly happy.

Social Pressures

As I started to write NOURISH, and as I began listening to mothers more intently, I noticed, quite surprisingly, that many of them had huge hang-ups about the same thing; namely being embarrassed, particularly at social events and gatherings, when wanting to say no to unhealthy foods. If this is you, then you are certainly not alone, and I implore you to try to think differently, especially if you are reading this and beginning to make significant lifestyle choices for your family. Do try to remember that if a high percentage of your child's food is prepared at home, and if you feel you are doing a good job there, then 'a little of something' won't go a long way to spoiling your child's appetite and health (or your efforts). Follow through with some of the strategies that I propose in this chapter and see how much easier they make it to say, 'No thank you' or 'Not now', or that will distract yourself and your children with other areas of play and enjoyment.

If that doesn't convince you, try thinking about it another way. When you attend an event your growing child will test you in many ways. Knowing whether certain foods are desirable or not won't be your only concern. Your child might take their pullover off when you know it's too cold to be without it, find a ginormous and highly dangerous stick and insist on waving it around, upset a friend or become upset... Every day, all day (as you well know) and not only at events, as a parent you are faced with the constant battle of trying to keep your child unharmed and happy. Why, then, should you feel embarrassed about steering your child away from food items that you know to have no beneficial gain when you instinctively guide them towards safe and healthy practices in so many other areas of their lives?

It is hard to stay healthy in some social situations, especially with my kids, so I relax a little. I'm still watching out for overly processed foods, especially those with colourings, but it's so hard to be one of the only mums who says no when so many tempting choices are around.
(Iona, mother to children aged eight and five)

One situation that I do find slightly more stressful and is sometimes more difficult to handle is when other people (other mums, parents or carers, who are caring and well intentioned) offer my children food without asking my permission. Again, this will depend on where you are living and the culture there, but some people think nothing of giving your child food. With Jul, of course, because of his allergies I had to be very careful of this, and over the years he would always come and ask me first. It isn't that easy for very small children, however, and I have regularly found my other two sons with food hanging out of their mouths. I really don't want to sound like a bore but I want to be the one who feeds my children – perhaps they are due for dinner and I don't want their appetite spoiled, or I simply don't want convenience, processed snacks (because that's what it generally is) given out without consideration. The way you are raising your child will help you respond to this situation and help you prevent conflict. Your child may feel frustrated, even upset that you disallow him something, especially if you have had to physically remove it after it's been given. Be firm and explain your reasons to your child. If it helps, perhaps you will offer your child something else from his or her own snack box.

Holidays

I appreciate that the time around holidays can be busy and often stressful, especially if you are travelling and staying for extended periods outside of the comforts of your family home. Adults during this time often forgo their health practices, surrendering nutritious food choices and exercise, and will very soon feel the consequences for doing so, generally gaining weight quickly and mainly just feeling out of sorts. While I realise that maintaining your regular routine will be difficult, it is really important to try as much as possible for your child. Try where viable not to let your child miss out on the nutrient-dense foods they are used to eating now, and while I realise that sugar-laden, overly processed foods will be more difficult to avoid, seek to find a compromise with your child that allows them to enjoy themselves and some of these foods without too much concern.

Food on the Go

If you find yourself in a situation where you do have to feed your family on a journey (and let's admit it, it can happen sometimes), if you are willing to go out of your way to look for it, I think you might agree, that for the most part, you can usually find something nutritious to eat.

There is no need to panic or assume too quickly that you won't be able to continue to feed your family well. Most restaurants are very accommodating if you ask for something simple or would like a recipe modified. In supermarkets that you pass along the way, you will find fresh produce, and even petrol stations offer a small selection of healthy choices.

Something to Think About

Being prepared will always be a better option when travelling though, so whenever possible make and pack your family a lunch box to take with you while you travel, especially if your journey means you would otherwise have to stop for meals. Not having to compromise over food options will save you the conflict you will likely encounter if your child has to choose from an array of less-than-adequate options.

Treats

As mothers it is typical to want to reward your child for good deeds and tasks well done, however it may become a problem if you do so with junk food. Giving your child food typically considered unhealthy can be unclear and confuse the child, leading them to negatively connect such foods with good behaviours. Instead, reward your child with stickers, or new paints, a day out at the local museum or zoo, alone time with Mum and Dad, or a play date for example. I am not saying that you will be able to avoid (or want to give up) ever offering your child convenience foods, but associating the times that you do as being 'special' or as a 'treat' is not recommended.

"Some time ago my Dad let me try cotton candy; it was my first time having it. I said, 'You're right, Dad, it's delicious when you eat it but then you want to barf!'
(Kieran, aged fifteen)

Remember that some of us crave foods simply because we are told, or tell ourselves, we cannot have them, and children are no different. If your child feels deprived or left out (from the 'treats' his or her friends are having), consider giving them something from time to time. I make sure to stock up on some simple, quality chocolate bars and organic lollipops, and regularly prepare fancy-looking (but nutritious) home-made cupcakes etc. If I feel like it, without any expectations, there will be times where I'll just offer them – I try to make no association with behaviours, and don't offer them as a dessert if only they have eaten their dinner, for example. I feel that by doing so my children have a healthy association with such foods. If this is something you would like to try, do where possible avoid confectionery that contains significant amounts of empty calories, added sugars, extra fat, saturated fats, and excess preservatives and artificial dyes.

Making a Change

I acknowledge that not everyone can understand or appreciate the importance I put on health and how that affects the way I raise my family. Some people may even feel threatened by the healthy eating and lifestyle choices that you are now choosing to make. Many may see this change as you being different, while others will respect and even admire your efforts – be prepared for all views. This can be very difficult to accept, but if you persevere, try to stay included and include others; there will be no need for social events to be awkward or difficult.

Live by Example

Where I live I am very fortunate to have so many others support me and raise their own children in much the same way. For me and my family, it's just our lifestyle now. Yet, in the past, I have been probed at parties as to why I don't give my children certain foods, persuaded to let my children have 'treats' and coaxed into buying unsuitable products, but no more. If I am questioned now over my family's healthy habits I simply try to convey the positivity that living this way has brought to each one of us.

> *It's easy for me to choose healthy foods as my mum educated herself when she was young. Without her I think it would be difficult.*
> *(Student, aged eight and a half)*

Something to Think About
Remember that the hard work you are putting in each and every day will mean that one event a week or so won't harm your child. Remember it is not what you do some of the time, but what you do most of the time that counts.

Strategies for Change:
- Offer to bring a dish to share at social gatherings – that way your child will recognise foods that he or she is used to, and can eat them in abundance (fruit or veggie kebabs are always a good, fun option that most children enjoy).
- Before an event, consider giving your child a good snack or meal, because after all you may not know at what time they will be fed. This way, not only will your child have the energy they need to play, but they are far less likely to overindulge in the unhealthy foods on offer.
- Be sure to help your child make the most of any social event. Remember it is the occasion that is special and not just the food.

Self-Preservation

I have seen it time and time again: how mothers go to great lengths to cherish and feed their children well, but totally neglect their own needs and eating habits in the process. Picture this (a true story): a pregnant mother wakes after a disturbed night's sleep, following regular coughing from her six-year-old, and her almost three-year-old wanting to use the loo. It is a school morning and so she starts to prepare not only the family's breakfast of freshly squeezed juice, fresh fruit and French toast, but the kids' packed lunches, sandwiches, boiled eggs, sliced cheese, fruit wedges and raisins. As she helps to ensure her children eat well, dress and get off to school on time, she feels the strain of the later stages of pregnancy. This mother, after two whole hours of being awake, has not consumed a single ounce of food, or worse, a single drop of water! Now absolutely ravenous for anything she can lay her hands on, she devours some leftover toast and opts for tea instead of fresh juice, and dashes on with the rest of her morning. (You might have already guessed that this was me!)

This is quite clearly not a great way to start your day, not an optimum breakfast for someone expending the amount of energy that I was, and certainly not a great role model, but nevertheless what might be a typical day in many of your households. Unless you make yourself a priority, and by that I mean practising the art of taking care of yourself, anything and everything will come before you and your needs.

Self-Worth and Importance

As a mother, it is so easy to put everything else first because everything *is* important. Children and their needs are particularly demanding at a young age, only adding to the energy and patience you need. It can feel like so much is happening all of the time, because it probably is!

I quickly learned as a mother that priorities change and everyone's demands and circumstances will be different. When Jul was ill, the priority in our family was doing everything we could to help him, but this also meant my husband and I taking care of each other and allowing help from others so that we had enough energy to care for him and go on with the other duties of life.

Eat Well

This guide and all that it contains is not meant to show you how much you are not doing, but to encourage you to reach out for support and when the going gets tough, admit that you may need some help. Putting yourself first is a must. Doing so will allow you to cope better with the stresses of motherhood and model healthy habits with conviction. The notion of doing something each and every day for yourself may take time, but below are some examples of small but realistic ways you can start.

> *I have learned to make it a priority to take care of myself. Like all the other important things I have to do in my day, I schedule the time to exercise, prepare foods and do a little something for myself. What's more, I think it's imperative that my children see me doing this.*
> *(Janice, mother to children aged sixteen, six and four)*

Do something Just for You

Before motherhood your schedule was probably filled with a lot of social engagements, evening get-togethers with your girlfriends, time carved out for the salon, and maybe a hobby or two. Fast-forward to motherhood and everything gets put on hold, which is totally normal and fine, that is, for an acceptable period of time. Making time just you for is essential to maintaining balance.

Find Reinforcement

Reach out to those family members, friends or peers who you can depend upon, and gain strength from each other. It can be frustrating to follow a certain way of life when those around you are following theirs in a different way, but trust in what you believe in and the steps you are taking for you and your family.

Relax

One really must make the time to relax by having some 'time off' from the demands of parenthood. That may sound like an impossible thing to accomplish, but by planning ahead at least one day in advance, you can surely make it work. Maybe you have family members or friends who can reliably allow you to take some time away from home? If not, then at the very least make the absolute most of when children are taking naps or when they go to bed at night. One of my favourite things to do is to close the bathroom door and have a nice hot bath.

4. Eat Well

It is so common during the months and years of early motherhood to neglect your eating habits. When you are tired and taking care of your precious baby or child, a lot of their needs will come first. To stay healthy, it is important for you to feed yourself and to do it well. If you allow your body to go too long without the essential nutrients, you will end up burnt out. Promise yourself that you will do better because you have earned it!

Firstly, when you have the time, stock the freezer with healthy meals, so you will have something nutritious at hand when you are hungry. Secondly, whether it's the father of your child or a significant other, it's important to let them know just how much their support and specifically their help in the kitchen, at this time, means to you. Thirdly, instead of having to find the time to shop when it is just too inconvenient for you or your child, have your produce home-delivered (if this is an option where you live). By doing so, you will have a kitchen stocked with healthy produce, which will invariably help you to avoid convenience foods.

5. Don't Multitask

Wow, once again this may sound contradictory to being a busy mum, but do we really ever get anything done faster by doing more than one thing at a time? The answer is likely no. You may feel as if you are being efficient but what you need to be is effective – there is a big difference.

> *As a mother I see myself as the core of my family, and because of that, I take my health very seriously. I notice that when I relax my rules the whole concept of what I have been trying to encourage just kind of crumbles. Since having my youngest daughter I have become even more passionate about building a healthy future for our family, even making it into a business, helping other women and moms alike. Having something else to focus on also allows me the time away, that as a strong and independent woman we all need and crave.*
> *(Heather, mother to daughters aged four and two)*

Strategies for Change:

- Believe in yourself. By acknowledging your own self-belief you give yourself permission to follow your passions and do what you really trust in, for both you and your family.
- If there are phases in your busy life where fitting in meals seems impossible, try snacking on well-balanced mini-meals to ensure your energy levels remain high.
- Consider stopping all chores at least thirty minutes before bedtime. As mothers this is imperative to winding down, falling asleep easily, and getting as much sleep as you can.

Professional's Comments: Vera Vergunst-Duijnhouwer MSc, Educational and Development Psychologist

Throughout this chapter I have spoken a lot about allowing a child to have autonomy. In your own words and experience, what is autonomy?

Autonomy is about your child feeling that they have the ability to influence their own life. To enhance this feeling of autonomy you should treat your child as an equal to you, with their own needs, emotions and desires. These needs will not always be in line with your own, and as parents, this is something important to comprehend.

How does autonomy work when, as parents, we are struggling to feed our children with options they don't always like?

By accepting your child's autonomy around food choices, you allow your child to feel comfortable around eating, something that is especially important as your child ages. Give your child the opportunity to pick foods, give them a range of healthy choices, but let them choose which of these they would like to eat, and also the amount of food they want to put on their plate etc. An example that I use in my own house is allowing my children to choose a menu for two or three nights every week. This is something that they can do on their own, to plan and look forward to, with very little input from me. A child with a feeling of autonomy will be much more open to your suggestions when you need them to cooperate (e.g. by eating a food or meal that is not their favourite), because he or she knows you will not force them into anything he or she doesn't genuinely want.

Is there anything more you would like us to know about autonomy?

Autonomy is linked to a 1970's theory called the self-determination theory (SDT). It is a philosophy that fosters three human psychological needs used in many, if not all areas of our life. According to current theorists Deci and Ryan (2000), these include:

Competence: seeking to control the outcome of an event, and to experience a level of mastery *(I can do this and I can do it on my own, and I can do it on my own well).*

Relatedness: a universal want to interact, to be connected to, and to experience caring for others *(I want to be involved, I want to be involved with others, I want to matter, I want to matter to others and have them matter to me).*

Autonomy: the urge to be the agent of one's own life.

If we relate this to the areas of health and wellness we might conclude that by giving our children the opportunity to learn competence, have relatedness and show autonomy, we are providing them with the motivation, self-taught skills and confidence to put into place healthy practices throughout their daily lives.

Nurture – Your Questions Answered

I'm concerned that my child is making unhealthy food choices when he is outside of the home, how can I prevent this from happening?

Even with the very best of intentions it will be difficult for your child, especially if you are not there and/or he is with his peers, to always make healthy choices. If you are genuinely doing all that you can to cultivate good food choices at home, and you see that your child is grasping the concept of why this is so important, then please allow him the freedom without your constant questioning when he is out of the house and with friends. I have been pleasantly surprised over the past few months as my own sons mature to see them choosing fresh juices where some of their friends choose sodas, refrain from asking for more sweets when they're offered, and only last weekend Jul called me up from a friend's birthday party to ask me if it was OK if he ate fast food from an outlet that we would not normally frequent. Of course my answer was yes, I didn't want him to feel left out, but I was so proud of him for checking with me and to my astonishment when he returned home he told me that he had not really enjoyed it. In my experience, when you provide your children with the opportunity to eat a diet that is truly sufficient, they seldom actually want or prefer anything else.

As a mother, I am dedicated to making changes that I know are beneficial for better health. However I don't feel supported by my family, what can I do?

It is typically the mother who shoulders the responsibility for feeding her family, and what you have probably found is that in the former years of your child's life, this was easy or at least easier than what you are experiencing now. Making changes to an already established way of eating can be difficult, and it is not uncommon for other family members to resist or rebel against this. In my personal experience, firstly you need to be the change that you want to see in others. It isn't enough for you to tell your family what to do or what to eat, it is essential however for you to show them, and to be a role model that they can look up to and emulate. Even my husband and I who struggle with eating healthy from time to time will admit that we do a lot better when the other is fostering habits that contribute to better well-being. Showing your family the way and being patient with change, will, in the long run, help them to adopt a healthier lifestyle.

Is my child's picky eating a result of nature or nurture?

Although there have been some very significant and convincing studies to show that the influence of genetic factors plays a part in whether or not a child will be a picky eater or have fussy tendencies, parents should not admit defeat. After all, your child still needs to eat and you need to find a way to help him do this without too much distraction or drama. Together with many other routines that you are following to help your growing child, you can positively influence eating behaviours through relatable modifications and constant reinforcement.

Resources and Recommendations

Some of the world's leading experts in food, health and wellness. Also some of my favourite, oh-so-inspiring, informative and reliable resources and tools.

Websites

Dreena Burton
www.plantpoweredkitchen.com
Best selling cookbook author, educator and mother to three girls, Dreena Burton shows us how effortlessly providing our families with plant-powered foods can enrich both our health and our lives.

Ella Mills
www.deliciouslyella.com
Ella became known for her popular blog that chronicled her journey from extreme sickness to vibrant health. Now a bestselling author, deli owner and entrepreneur, Ella shows us how health in all areas of our lives is possible.

Environmental Working Group
www.ewg.com
A non-profit organisation, their mission is *to empower people to live healthier lives in a healthier environment with breakthrough research and education.* Take a look at their consumer guides that will help you to find the safest products from food sources to sunscreen. No matter where you live in the world, these resources will be invaluable.

Food Matters®
www.foodmatters.com
Uncovers the secrets of natural health to help you achieve optimum wellness!

Jamie Oliver
www.jamieoliver.com
Celebrity chef, restaurateur and cookbook author, Jamie Oliver has done remarkable work to help bring about awareness and change in school food across the UK.

Joel Fuhrman MD
www.drfuhrman.com
A family doctor, for over twenty-five years, Dr Fuhrman helps people sustain good health through his philosophy of nutritional medicine. Dr Fuhrman is also an author, speaker and popular media personality.

John Douillard
www.lifespa.com
Ayurvedic practitioner, author, leading alternative expert in health and wellness and father to six children, Douillard helps you to understand the importance of eating with the seasons and other Ayurvedic practices to assist you and your family towards a healthier lifestyle.

John Robbins
www.johnrobbins.info
The only heir to the Baskin-Robbins ice cream empire, Robbins decided to take a different path and pursue health. As an author and activist Robbins makes the connection between environmentalism, nutrition and animal rights.

Joshua Rosenthal
www.integrativenutrition.com
The found of the Institute for Integrative Nutrition, Joshua Rosenthal works passionately to educate individuals around the globe on the fundamentals of health and wellness.

Kris Carr
www.kriscarr.com
Founder of the Crazy Sexy Cancer wellness revolution. Inspiring, educational and always fun, Carr is a *New York Times* bestselling author, wellness advocate and cancer survivor, showS you how to lead an amazing, full and healthy life through the foods you eat.

Mark Hyman
www.drhyman.com
Dr Hyman, physician, scholar and *New York Times* bestselling author, comments, *Your fork, the most powerful tool to transform your health and change the world.*

Books

Joel Furhman: *Super Immunity*
John Douillard: *The 3-Season Diet* and *Perfect Health for Kids*
John Douillard: *Perfect Health for Kids*
Joshua Rosenthal: *Integrative Nutrition*
T. Colin Campbell: *The China Study*

Documentaries

Cowspiracy
Food, Inc.
Forks Over Knives
Sustainable
Two Angry Moms

Kitchen Appliances

Dehydrator: *Excalibur*
Food Processor: *Magimix*
High Speed Performance Blender: *Vitamix TNC*
Juicer: *Green Star*
KitchenAid: *Kenwood*

Products

I am in no way currently paid to endorse these products! Also check out The Environmental Working Group and their consumer guides for other essential products in and around your home.

Child's Farm
www.childsfarm.com
I recently came across this highly awarded UK brand and I am loving the bath and hair products for my boys. They claim to go above and beyond the standard EU regulations for testing of their products… I really like what this company stands for.

Dr Bronner

www.drbronner.co.uk

I have been using Dr Bronner bar soaps for many, many years now and love all of their scents. Their products are made from pure vegetable oils, are free from synthetic detergents, biodegradable, eco-friendly and fair trade. Dr Bronner's Baby Mild pure, unscented, organic bar soap is a good first addition to your baby or young child's routine.

Green People

www.greenpeople.co.uk

I choose Green People products for my children's oral hygiene because they like the flavours and I like the results they give. Different products are available for baby and child, so lots for you to choose from.

Trukid

www.trukid.com

My friends and I agree that the Sunny Days Daily 30 SPF+ sunscreen performs really well for our children, even those with sensitive skin.

Weleda

www.weleda.co.uk

Love, love, love all their mother and baby products, but particularly beneficial for my boys' skin (and recommended to so many of my friends too) is Baby Calendula Oil which you can add to damp skin every evening after a bath or shower. Even if you cannot purchase these products easily, check online and on Amazon, and if you have to (and can), have them shipped overseas. You won't regret it.

Work With Me

When was the last time you talked with an experienced professional about yourself and your health, and received the personal attention you deserve?

It's rare for anyone to get the chance they really crave to share their nutrition and wellness concerns. As a unique health counsellor, I create a supportive environment that will enable you to uncover and achieve both your short- and long-term goals.

Most approaches to nutrition dwell on strict guidelines that can lead to deprivation, making you feel anxious and alone. Instead of restrictions, I coach my clients to create a happy, healthy life in a way that is flexible, fun and free of denial and discipline.

No one programme works for everyone.

I will guide you to find the right programme that includes making food and lifestyle choices that best support who you are in your current life. This personalised plan and support will help you to make gradual, lifelong changes that will enable you to attain success.

As a client of my current health counselling programme, you will...

- Learn how to be more health-aware.
- Receive up-to-date nutrition education.
- Set and accomplish goals in a way that is empowering and exciting.
- Uncover truths about the food and health industries.
- Learn about new foods and how you can easily incorporate them into your diet.
- Learn how to maintain a diet that is unique to you and your needs.
- Understand what the body really needs.
- Increase energy levels.
- Introduce and incorporate non-traditional methods
- Discover the confidence to create the life you want for yourself and your family.
- ...And so much more!

To decide if health counselling is right for you (and your family), make an initial one-hour appointment. During this session, we will discuss your main concerns and how best I can support you.

For more information please visit
www.henryshealth.com

About the Author

Tamar Henry grew up in Bedfordshire, England, with her mother, father, older sister and younger brother. Through a series of work opportunities that saw Tamar travel the world, she met and married her husband. Together, they have three sons.

Tamar has a Bachelor of Science in health and wellness and is a certified holistic health and nutrition counsellor from the Institute for Integrative Nutrition (IIN).

She currently works as a health and nutrition counsellor in her community, and as the health and wellness advisor in a local primary school.

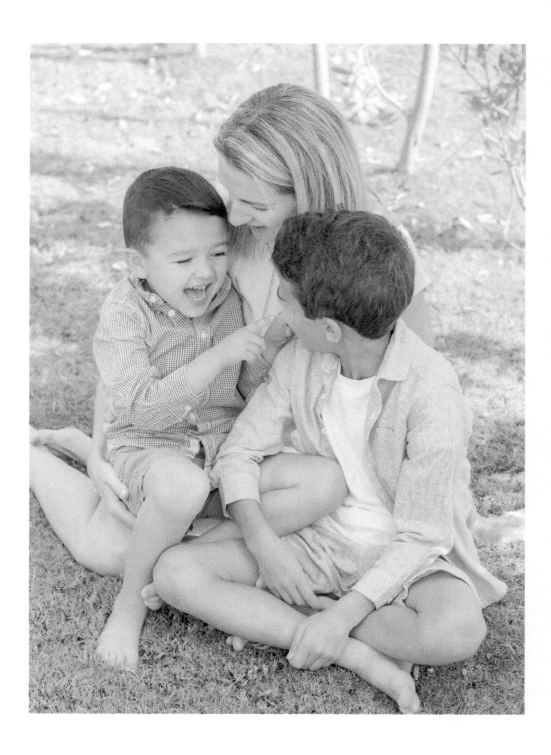